The Application of

RADIOIODINATED ROSE BENGAL AND COLLOIDAL RADIOGOLD

In the Detection of

HEPATOBILIARY DISEASE

A Monograph in
MODERN CONCEPTS OF RADIOLOGY, NUCLEAR MEDICINE
AND ULTRASOUND

Edited by

LEWIS E. ETTER, M.D., F.A.C.R.

Professor of Radiology
Western Psychiatric Institute
and Falk Clinic
Presbyterian-University Hospital
School of Medicine
University of Pittsburgh
Pittsburgh, Pennsylvania

The Application of

RADIOIODINATED ROSE BENGAL AND COLLOIDAL RADIOGOLD

In the Detection of

HEPATOBILIARY DISEASE

By

LEONARD ROSENTHALL, M.S., M.D.

Senior Radiologist and
Director of The Division of Nuclear Medicine
Montreal General Hospital
Associate Professor of Radiology
McGill University
Montreal, Canada

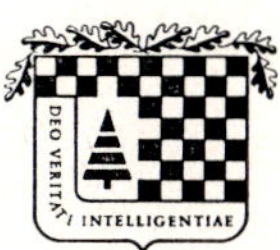

W A R R E N   H.   G R E E N ,   I N C.
St. Louis, Missouri, U.S.A.

Published by

WARREN H. GREEN, INC.
10 South Brentwood Blvd.
St. Louis, Missouri 63105, U.S.A.

Printed in the United States of America
5-B

DEDICATION

The author wishes to dedicate this monograph to his three paediatric liabilities: Wendy, Gary and Sandy, without whose help this might have been completed in half the time.

The author also wishes to dedicate this monograph to his wife, Devorah, without whose help this might have been completed in twice the time.

ACKNOWLEDGEMENTS

The author wishes to express his gratitude to the attending and resident staff of The Montreal General Hospital who were most cooperative in supporting the investigation of radiopharmaceuticals in the detection of hepatobiliary dysfunction. Appreciation of the contributions made by the members of the Department of Medical Illustration, and Chief Technician of the Division of Nuclear Medicine, Miss Judy Tremblay, R.T. (D., T., N.M.), must also be mentioned. A special thanks is due Mrs. Evelyn J. Whitaker for her patient and diligent preparation of the manuscript.

L. R.

CONTENTS

The Application of

RADIOIODINATED ROSE BENGAL AND COLLOIDAL RADIOGOLD

In the Detection of

HEPATOBILIARY DISEASE

Chapter 1

PHYSIOLOGY OF ROSE BENGAL

Rose bengal is a fluorescent dye. It is the potassium or sodium salt of tetrachlorotetraiodofluorescein (Fig. 1-1), and was first

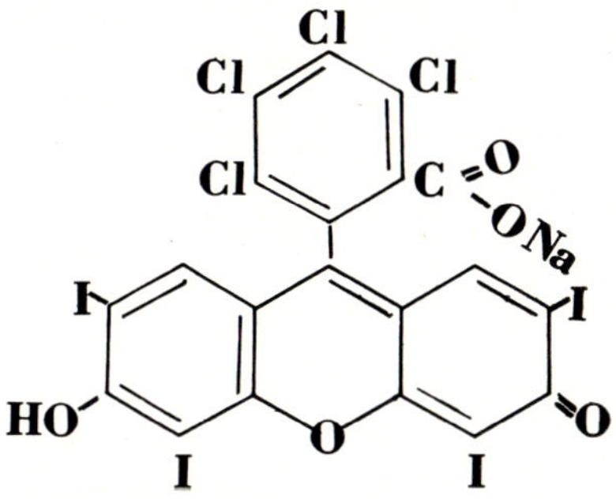

FIGURE 1-1.   Sodium salt of tetrachlorotetraiodofluorescein.

reported as a useful agent to determine the functional state of the liver colorimetrically in 1923 (1). The dye is rapidly removed from the blood stream almost entirely by the parenchymal cells of the liver and excreted into the bile. It flows with the bile into the gall bladder and duodenum, and there is virtually complete recovery in the stool.

Mendeloff (2) utilized the fluorescent property of rose bengal to depict histologically its location in the polygonal rather than Kupffer cells of the liver in 1949. Studies on the extrahepatic clearance of rose bengal by Sapirstein and Simpson in 1955 (3) showed no staining of the abdominal organs other than the liver and gall bladder, even after prolonged infusion of the dye.

Introduction of radioactive iodine (^{131}I) into the rose bengal molecule by Taplin *et al.* (4, 5) in 1954 permitted further evaluation of its physiological properties. To determine which liver cell concentrated the dye the reticuloendothelial system of rabbits was blocked with numerous agents. These included colloidal thorium dioxide, india ink, hcmolized erythrocytes and gelatin. A number of animals received 1,000 r whole body irradiation in 7 to 10 days. Although phagocytic function of the reticuloendothelial system was shown to be significantly depressed in such irradiated or blocked livers, none of the animals exhibited abnormal radioactive rose bengal liver uptake or excretion patterns. In another series of experiments, they instilled a given quantity of radioiodinated rose bengal into the duodenum of rabbits following intubation and could not detect activity in the liver either with external counting over the organ or tissue assay. This indicated that the aqueous solution of rose bengal is not absorbed from the gut. To show that the rose bengal elaborated by the liver and mixed with bile is also not absorbed from the bowel, one rabbit was intravenously injected with ^{131}I rose bengal and the bile was shunted from the duodenum of this animal into the duodenum of a second rabbit. Again, no activity was exhibited in the liver of the second animal.

Jacobson and Brent (6) investigated the distribution of ^{131}I rose bengal in the rat in relation to time. They showed by tissue assay that the amount of ^{131}I accumulated by the thyroid considerably exceeded the quantity expected from the free ^{131}I in the rose bengal solution at the time of injection. A similar *in vivo* dissociation of ^{131}I from the rose bengal molecule was demonstrated in man in a patient with biliary atresia. These same authors administered ^{131}I rose bengal directly into the stomach of several rats and found, by tissue assay, amounts of activity in the liver and thyroid that were higher than elsewhere in the carcass. This suggestion of intestinal absorption, albeit to a small extent, of intact ^{131}I rose bengal and dissociated ^{131}I is at variance with Taplin *et al.* (4, 5).

Delprat (1) could find no evidence of rose bengal excretion in the urine. Jacobson and Brent (6) showed that 5% of the intravenously administered ^{131}I rose bengal appeared in the urine of the rat in approximately forty-five hours, most of this in the first 24 hours. Sutherland (14) has shown qualitatively that rose bengal is excreted in the urine both in normal and abnormal patients. Additional work is necessary to sort out the amount of free ^{131}I, ^{131}I- rose bengal and unlabeled rose bengal in the urine in relation to surgical and medical jaundice.

Lushbough *et al.* (7) observed the elimination of ^{131}I rose bengal in normal subjects with a large whole body liquid scintillation well counter (8). The retention curve obtained consisted of two exponential components with half-times of 18 hours and 50 days. The latter corresponded to the urinary excretion rate of iodine which was organified by the thyroid and bound to the hormonal iodine pool.

An extensive study on the distribution and kinetics of ^{131}I rose bengal was carried out by Meurman (9). He found by chromatographic analysis that the stable and radioactive rose bengal consisted of 7 to 10 components. An analysis of the serum-dye mixture showed that the main part of the radioactive dye combined with albumin and contained 75% of the activity. The rest was distributed evenly among the globulin fractions, but it was felt that there was probably some albumin absorbed in the globulin area of the electrophoretic strip, and very little activity was attached to the globulin. Chromatography of ^{131}I rose bengal excreted into the bile showed that the different fractions were all recovered in approximately the same proportions as they occurred in the injected material.

Bocci (10) was able to isolate one of the fractions of ^{131}I rose bengal with paper chromatography. The component contained 41% of the total radioactivity and no free ^{131}I. The blood decay curve obtained in rabbits was precisely the same as when using the original multi-component labelled rose bengal, i.e., approximately bi-exponential. It was concluded that the shape of the rose bengal plasma curve was not due to the heterogenerity of dyes, but solely to the biological situation. Samples of rabbit bile collected at different times following injection of labelled rose bengal were subjected to ascending paper chromatography, and there was no evidence of transformation or conjugation of the dye.

An autoradiographic study in rats (9) depicted a centrilobular concentration of ^{131}I rose bengal in the liver. Fifteen to 24 hours after the bile duct was obstructed, the autoradiograms showed a more uniform distribution between the centrilobular zones and periportal areas.

On the other hand, Glasser *et al.* (11) state that the auto-radiograms of livers from rats killed at two minutes show that the dye had already spread through the entire parenchyma, but with a higher concentration around the portal triads, and lesser amounts in the region of the central veins. It would appear that this minor problem is not resolved as yet.

The kinetics of ^{131}I rose bengal has been studied by a number of investigators by compartmental analysis (7, 9, 12, 13). Most of the difficulties arise from the fact that extrahepatic routes of clearance are only partially known, and the effects of polygonal cell impairment and bile obstruction on these routes are even less understood.

BIBLIOGRAPHY

1. DELPRAT, G. D.: Studies on liver function: Rose bengal elimination from the blood as influenced by liver injury. *Arch. Int. Med.,* *32*:401, 1923.
2. MENDELOFF, A. I.: Fluorescence of intravenously administered rose bengal appears only in polygonal cells. *Proc. Soc. Exper. Biol. &* *Med., 70*:556, 1949.
3. SAPIRSTEIN, L. A., AND SIMPSON, A. M.: Plasma clearance of rose bengal (tetraiodotetrabromfluorescein). *Am. J. Physiol., 182*:337, 1955.
4. TAPLIN, G. V., MEREDITH, O. M., AND KADE, H.: The Radioactive (^{131}I tagged) Rose Bengal Uptake Excretion Test for Liver Function using external Gamma-ray Scintillation Counting Techniques. USAEC Report UCLA-319, University of California at Los Angeles, 1954.
5. TAPLIN, G. V., MEREDITH, O. M., AND KADE, H.: The radioactive (I^{131} tagged) rose bengal uptake excretion test for liver function using external gamma-ray scintillation counting techniques. *J. Lab. Clin. Med., 45*:665, 1955.
6. JACOBSON, A. G., AND BRENT, R. L.: The fate of I^{131} tagged rose bengal

in the rat. *Am. J. of Roentgenol., Rad. Therapy & Nuclear Medicine,* 79:1004, 1958.

7. LUSHBAUGH, C. C., KRETCHMAN, A., AND GIBBS, W.: Liver function measured by the blood clearance of rose bengal -I^{131}: A review and a model based on compartmental analysis of changes in arm, blood, and liver radioactivity. In, *Dynamic Clinical Studies with Radioisotopes,* pages 319-357. Edited by R. M. Kniseley, W. N. Tauxe and E. B. Anderson. Published by the U. S. Atomic Energy Commission, Division of Technical Information.

8. ANDERSON, E. C., SCHUCH, R. L., PERRINGS, J. D., AND LANGHAM, W. H.: The Los Alamos human counter. *Nucleonics, 14*(1):26, 1956.

9. MEURMAN, L.: On the distribution and kinetics of injected I^{131} rose bengal. An experimental study with special reference to the evaluation of liver function. *Acta Med. Scand., 167,* Suppl. 354, 1960.

10. BOCCI, V.: Distribution and fate of rose bengal. *Nature, 189*:584, 1961.

11. GLASSER, W., GIBBS, W. D., AND ANDREWS, G. A.: The mechanism of removal of rose bengal from the plasma of the rat. *J. Lab. and Clin. Med., 54*:556, 1959.

12. DORLEYN, M., AND COENEGRACHT, J.: Quantitative measurement of liver function with radioactive rose bengal. *Medicamundi, 5*:35, 1959.

13. TURCO, G. L., GEHEMI, F., MOLINO, G., AND SEGRE, G.: The kinetics of I^{131} rose bengal in normal and cirrhotic subjects studied by compartmental analysis and a digital computer. *J. Lab. Clin. Med.,* 7:983, 1966.

14. SUTHERLAND, J. B.: Personal communication. Winnipeg General Hospital, Winnipeg, Man.

Chapter 2

RADIOIODINATED ROSE BENGAL CLEARANCE AS A TEST OF HEPATOBILIARY FUNCTION

THE COLORIMETRIC ROSE bengal test of liver damage has received relatively little attention compared to bromsulfalein since its introduction in 1923, in spite of a series of papers between 1923 and 1933 demonstrating its effectiveness (1, 2, 3, 4, 5, 6). A general feeling pervaded many institutions that the test was not as sensitive as the bromsulfalein study, and the latter therefore received more investigative attention and was much more widely publicized. This was abetted by a comparative analysis of the two dyes in 24 non-jaundiced patients with liver disease which was published in 1949 by Monroe and Hopper (7). They found that 41% of the patients with normal rose bengal tests had positive bromsulfalein determinations, and concluded the latter was more sensitive as measured by the visual spectrograph. Very little, pro or con, appeared in the literature after that report until Taplin and his associates introduced [131]I- labelled rose bengal in 1954 (8, 9). This initiated a flurry of activity which resulted in both favorable and unfavorable communications as to its efficacy as an indicator of hepatic damage. Much attention was paid to analyzing the liver uptake-excretion curves obtained by placing an external scintillation detector probe over the liver and recording on a strip chart the activity versus time following an intravenous injection of [131]I- rose bengal. Characteristic curves for various hepatobiliary aberrations such as acute hepatitis, chronic hepatitis, partial biliary obstruction and complete biliary

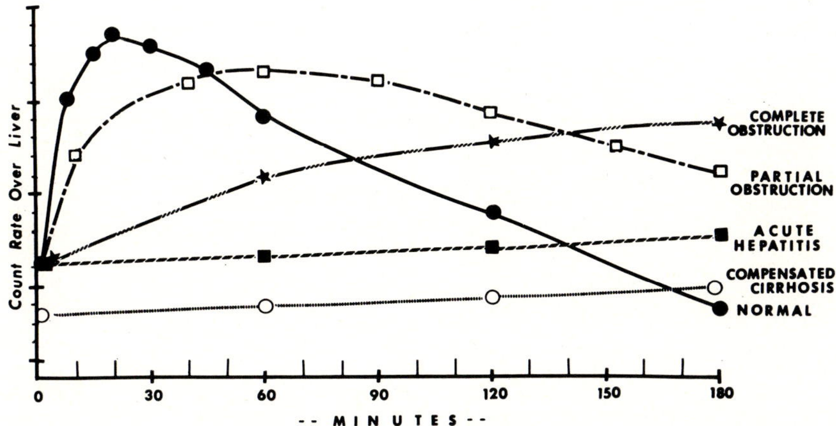

FIGURE 2-1. Compilation of schematic curves of [131]I- rose bengal liver uptake in a variety of hepatobiliary disorders.

obstruction were reported (10). Figure 2-1 is a compilation of schematic curves obtained in a variety of conditions.

LIVER UPTAKE—EXCRETION ANALYSIS

The validity of the radioactive rose bengal uptake-excretion curves obtained by external counting was studied in 14 cholecystectomized patients by Engler *et al.* (11). A correlation coefficient of 0.9 was obtained between the rate of removal of activity from the plasma and the hepatic uptake, and also between the rate of accumulation of activity of aspirated bile and hepatic excretion. This suggested a one-to-one relationship between the respective parameters with regard to rose bengal economy.

The uptake-excretion curves obtained over the liver were analyzed in 18 normal subjects, 12 patients with polygonal cell jaundice, and 6 patients with obstructive jaundice by Cohn *et al.* (12). A high degree of variability was observed in the maximum peak of the curve, the time required to reach maximum peak, and the height of the curve at each fifteen minute interval following the injection of radioactive dye in both normals and icteric patients. The patterns were stated to be not significantly consistent or definitive to distinguish parenchymous and obstructive jaundice. Part of the difficulty lay in the positioning of the probe where a slight tilt resulted in a considerable variation in count rate. This was due to any combination of factors such as radioactive dye in the gall bladder, biliary tree, duodenum and blood.

Brown and Glasser (13) also found the qualitative analysis of liver uptake-excretion curves unreliable. They could find a significant difference between a cirrhotic group and normals, but not between the cirrhotics and those with obstruction. A suggestion that the amount of bilirubin present in the polygonal cell in obstructive jaundice interferes with rose bengal uptake was refuted by Taplin *et al.* (10), who found no alteration in ^{131}I- rose bengal uptake when serum bilirubin levels were raised a hundredfold experimentally in rabbits.

Lowenstein (14) attempted to analyze the liver curves mathematically. The tracing was transcribed onto semi-logarithmic paper, and the descending portion of the curve was extrapolated back as a straight line to intersect the ordinate at Eo. By subtracting the liver curve from this excretion line, another straight line is obtained, the uptake line, which intersects the ordinate at Uo (Fig. 2-2). The following results were reported by Lowenstein (15):

	Uptake Half Time (Uo/2) In Minutes	Excretion Half Time (Eo/2) In Hours
Normal	9	1.5
Laennec's Cirrhosis	18	5
Biliary Cirrhosis	28	24
Obstructive Jaundice	15	24

Moertel and Owen (16) used the Lowenstein analysis of the radioactive rose bengal uptake-excretion tracings over the liver in non-jaundiced patients with hepatocellular damage. A concomitant bromsulfalein study was made. They found that the average rate of hepatic uptake of the radioactive dye was slower in patients with hepatic disease than it was in control subjects, but a large overlap occurred between the individual values of the group with liver disease and the control group. They could not recommend the radioactive rose bengal test because of this lack of sensitivity in non-jaundiced patients with liver disease, and the one to two hours required for its performance. In plot-

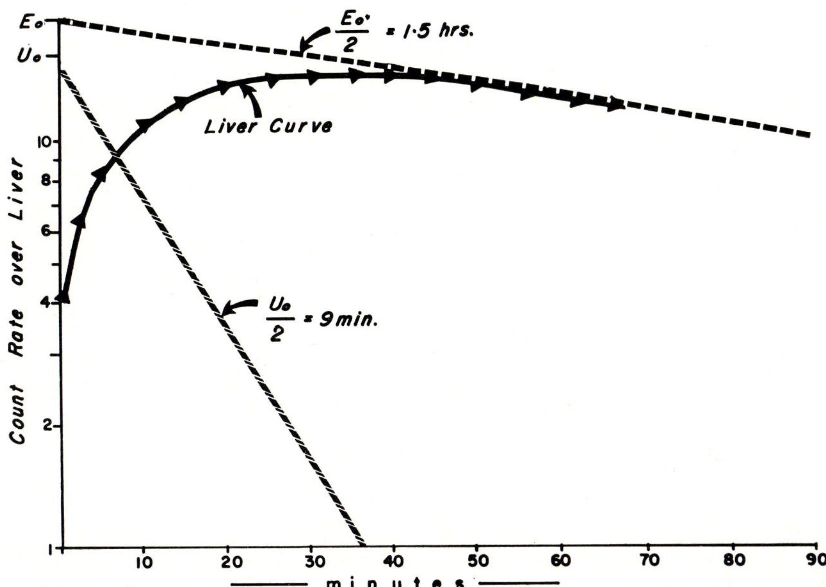

FIGURE 2-2. Lowenstein analysis of the [131]I- rose bengal liver uptake curve. The uptake half-time (Uo/2) is 9 minutes, and the excretion half-time (Eo/2) is 1.5 hours for this normal schematic curve.

ting the radioactive rose bengal values against the bromsulfalein retentions in those patients who had a variety of hepatic disorders such as cirrhosis, metastatic tumour, hemochromatosis, ctc., it was found that the mean uptake half time (Uo/2) of ^{131}I-rose bengal tends to increase as the retention of bromsulfalein increases. However, considerable overlap occurs between values in the normal group and in groups with minimal, and even pronounced, retention of bromsulfalein.

Richman and Jacobs (17) also found that monitoring the liver uptake and excretion of [131]I- rose bengal did not help characterize any type of hepatocellular disease, nor distinguish polygonal cell and obstructive jaundice, even when subjected to Lowenstein's mathematical analysis.

Another approach to liver monitoring of rose bengal uptake and excretion was proposed by Westover *et al.* (18). With the patient lying supine, the detector is placed anterolaterally over the liver at the 8th or 9th rib interspace. A small dose of ^{131}I-human serum albumin (about 2 microcuries) is intravenously administered, and the liver activity is recorded on a strip chart for two to three minutes until a plateau is sustained. An equal dose of ^{131}I- rose bengal is injected and recorded on the same strip chart. The fraction of activity within the liver blood pool taken up by the polygonal cells per minute (Q) is determined by the relationship:

$$Q = \frac{At_2 - At_1}{Vp\,(t_2 - t_1)}$$

Where, At_2 is the count rate at 10 minutes after injection of ^{131}I- rose bengal.

        At_1 is the count rate 3 minutes after injection of ^{131}I- rose bengal.

        Vp is the count rate of the plateau obtained with ^{131}I- human serum albumin, and thus reflects the liver blood pool of ^{131}I- rose bengal, since equal doses of both test agents are used.

In normal individuals, the value of Q is between 11% and 20% per minute. The authors admit that the determination will not always separate cases where a difference in hepatic function actually exists.

Lum and associates (19) combined liver monitoring with blood samples. A standard dose of 5 microcuries ^{131}I- rose bengal containing 5 grams of stable dye was administered via vena puncture. When the tracing over the liver reached its peak a 1 ml blood sample was drawn and counted in a well counter. Liver counts and blood sample assays were repeated at 6 and 24 hours. They derived the following scheme to differentiate jaundice.

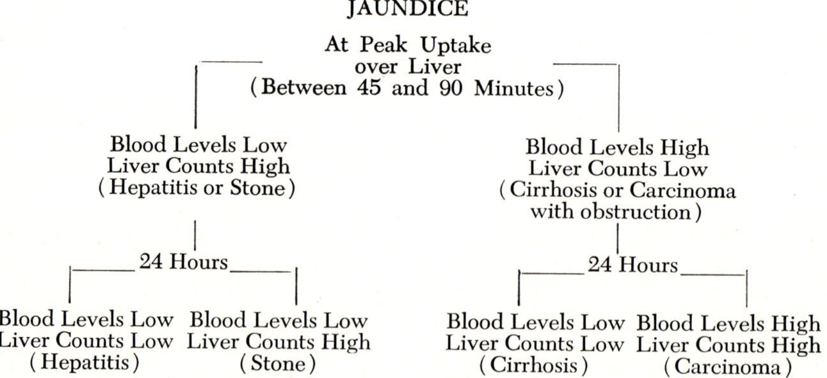

Still another variation of the liver monitoring technique of radioiodinated rose bengal uptake was presented by Kawaguchi *et al.* (20, 21). Continuous counts are obtained over the liver and abdomen following an intravenous dose of 10 to 15 microcuries. Approximately 45 minutes afterward the patient is given sodium dehydrocholate intravenously and 0.6 mg of nitroglycerin sublingually. Ten minutes later another 0.6 mg. of nitroglycerin is offered. Liver and abdomen recording continue for an additional 45 minutes, i.e., for a total of 90 minutes.

Liver uptake (LU) is calculated from the following relationship:

$$LU\ (\%/\text{min.}) = \frac{(\text{Count rate at 7 minutes})\quad\text{minus}\quad(\text{count rate at 2 minutes})}{(\text{Count rate at 1 minute})\quad\text{times}\quad(\text{5 minutes})}$$

where the count rate at 1 minute reflects the liver blood pool.

Intestinal entry (IE) is defined as:

$$IE\ (\%/\text{min.}) = \frac{\text{Maximum count rate over the abdomen after dehydrocholate and nitroglycerin}}{\text{Count rate over abdomen 2 minutes after }^{131}\text{I- rose bengal administration}}$$

An analysis of normal subjects, and jaundiced and non-jaundiced patients with a variety of hepatobiliary disorders yielded the following general results.

	LU	IE	IE/LU
Normal	19-37%	250-531%	—
Hepatocellular disease	Less than 19%	Less than 250%	Greater than 17
Extrahepatic obstruction (non-malignant)	Less than 19%	Less than 250%	Less than 17

The differentiation of intrahepatic and extrahepatic obstruction was difficult.

LIVER AND ARM MONITORING

A comprehensive analysis of the results obtained by monitoring the ^{131}I- rose bengal liver uptake, and arm and blood disappearance was published by Lushbaugh, Kretchmar and Gibbs (22). Their experiments were initiated to test the sensitivity of radioactive rose bengal in detecting minimal degrees of polygonal cell dysfunction. An external scintillation detector was carefully placed over the liver, and the patient's arm was inserted into the well of a liquid scintillation counter. The data from both devices were recorded continuously on a strip chart. A dose of 10 microcuries of ^{131}I rose bengal containing 0.06 to 2.4 mg of dye was administered intravenously, and the activity levels were recorded for 90 to 120 minutes. (Taplin *et al.* (9) had previously shown the range of carrier dye used in this investigation did not affect the results of the test.) The arm clearance curves in normal subjects reached a lower level than the group with a small degree of hepatic dysfunction. A semi-logarithmic plot of the tracings revealed two exponential components. The faster segment had a half time of 7.5 ± 1.3 minutes in the controls, and 8.0 ± 1.2 minutes in the group with hepatic dysfunction. Respective values of 284 ± 166 minutes and 401 ± 249 minutes were derived for the slower component. These values do not show a significant disparity between the two test groups. However, the index of function, Uo/Eo, where Uo is the ordinate value at time zero of the fast component, and Eo is the corresponding value of the slower component, did give a good separation. In the normal group, Uo/Eo was 6.1 ± 0.87, and 1.7 ± 0.7 for the minimally afflicted patients. Other parameters such as clearance capacity and saturation time, which were derived by some debatable mathematical manoeuvers of the arm and liver curves, also gave better results than the half times of the fast and slow components of the arm clearance curves.

BROMSULFALEIN STRESS TESTING

A group of patients presumed to be free of liver disease was given both bromsulfalein and stable rose bengal simultaneously to determine the influence each has on the other's clearance (23). It was found by colorimetric measurement that bromsulfalein has a greater inhibitory effect on the removal of rose bengal from the blood stream than rose bengal has on bromsulfalein removal. This confirmed the earlier work of Mendeloff (24), and was later appreciated by Taplin and his associates (10), who measured the effect of bromsulfalein on the blood disappearance and liver uptake of simultaneously administered radioactive rose bengal.

Mena and co-workers (25) found that a dose of 5 mg/kg of bromsulfalein diminished the uptake of rose bengal to an abnormal range in 100% of the patients with liver disease tested, and in 48% of the normal controls. It was also found that 2.5 mg/kg of bromsulfalein depressed the uptake of rose bengal in the presence of liver disease, but did not affect normal individuals. They conducted their examination by prestressing the liver with 2.5 mg/kg bromsulfalein, then injected 0.03 microcuries/kg ^{131}I-human serum albumin while the liver was monitored with an external scintillation detector. When the curve reached a plateau 0.03 microcuries [131]I- rose bengal was administered and the count rate was recorded for an additional 10 minutes. The liver uptake was calculated from the following relationship:

$$\frac{(\text{10-minute count rate}) \ \text{minus} \ (\text{3-minute count rate})}{(\text{Count rate of the plateau attained with } [131]\text{I albumin}) \ \text{times} \ (\text{7 minutes})}$$

Normal values varied 11 to 20% per minute.

BLOOD SAMPLE ASSAY

Dyrbye and Christensen (26) found the radioactive rose bengal test a sensitive indicator of hepatic function. They used about 10 microcuries with 2.2 mg rose bengal carrier, and took blood samples at 3 and 20 minutes. The retention expressed as the percentage of the count rate at 20 minutes to 3 minutes ranged between 10 and 30% in normal subjects. A half disappearance time was also calculated, and a normal range of 5.2 to 8 minutes was obtained. A comparative study with bromsulfalein was not pursued.

Virtually no trace of the radioactive dye was found in the blood at 24 hours in normal individuals by Ackerman and McFee (27). The liver was also observed to retain enough function in polygonal cell damage and partial extrahepatic obstruction to clear the blood of radioactive rose bengal in this interval. However, in complete obstruction some residual activity was present. For a given dose of test agent, the amount of rose bengal in the blood at 24 hours in patients with complete extrahepatic obstruction exceeded the values obtained in partial obstruction and polygonal cell damage by a factor of 1.6 to 28.

HEAD MONITORING OF RADIOACTIVE
ROSE BENGAL REMOVAL

Blahd and Nordyke (28, 29) investigated in depth the idea of monitoring the head to observe the disappearance of ^{131}I rose bengal and its correlation with the type of underlying hepatic dysfunction. The external scintillation detector is placed over the temporal area, encompassing the ear, and following an injection of 10-25 microcuries of activity containing 0.1 to 1.0 mg rose bengal the count rate is recorded continually. The ratio of the net count rate at 20 minutes to the net count rate at 5 minutes was defined as the "20-minute retention" (Fig. 2-3A).

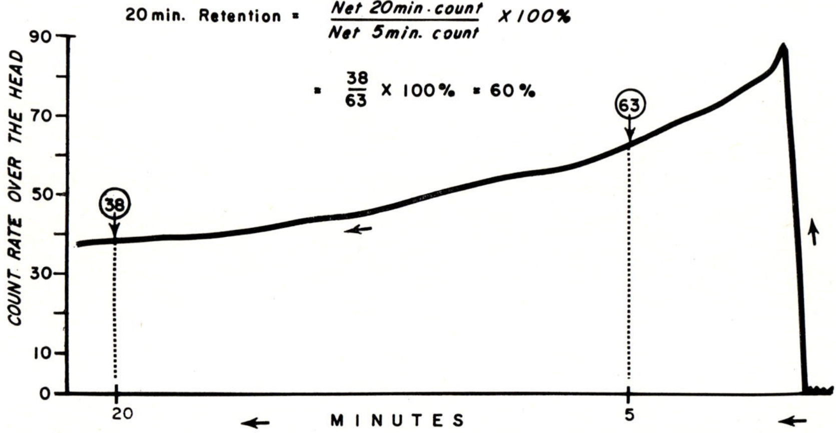

FIGURE 2-3A. ^{131}I- rose bengal disappearance curve of a patient with mild hepatocellular disease obtained by placing an external scintillation detector against the side of the head encompassing the ear. The 20-minute ^{131}I- rose bengal retention is a ratio of the net 20-minute count rate to the net 5-minute count rate.

The value of this index ranges between 39 to 51% in normal individuals. Retentions greater than 51% reflect polygonal cell disease and/or reduced perfusion of the liver. A retention exceeding 90% is virtually pathognomonic of primary hepatocellular disease, except where a prolonged complete obstruction is associated with pyrexia (30).

To distinguish extrahepatic and intrahepatic obstruction, Nordyke and Blahd (31) placed a second scintillation detector

over the abdomen in the left lower quadrant. The decline in the
head and abdomen tracings are parallel until the radioactive rose
bengal excreted by the liver enters the field of view of the
(Fig. 2-3B). Cholecystokinin is given intravenously 30 minutes

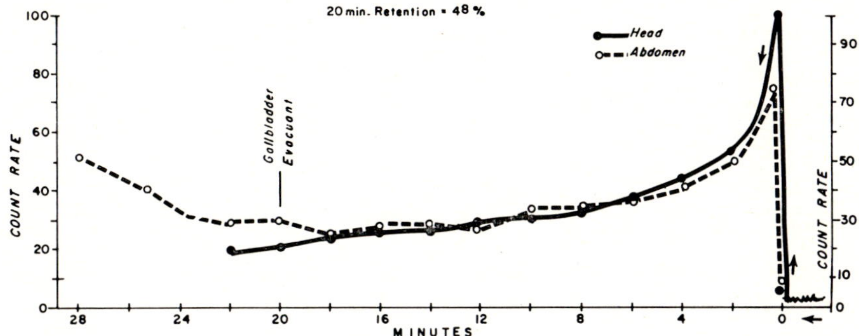

FIGURE 2-3B. ^{131}I- rose bengal curves obtained by placing external scintillation detectors against the head and over the left lower quadrant of the
abdomen in a normal patient. The head and abdomen tracings are parallel
until radioactive dye enters the bowel via the biliary system. A gall bladder
evacuant enhances the intestinal accumulation by contracting the gall
bladder.

after the ^{131}I- rose bengal to contract the gall bladder, relax the
sphincter of Oddi and cause any radioactive dye in the lower
biliary passages to flow into the bowel (30). If radioactivity is
observed in the gut within 15 minutes following administration
of cholecystokinin, the biliary tree was considered patent. A
second dose of cholecystokinin was given when activity was
not detected. Complete biliary tract obstruction was concluded
if the second attempt failed to reveal excretion into the gut.
Four categories are defined:

I	Normal	Retention less than 51% and prompt excretion into the gut in response to cholecystokinin.
II	Non-surgical jaundice	(a) Retention greater than 70% and slow but positive response to cholecystokinin. (b) Almost pathognomonic if retention is 90% or more.
III	Surgical Jaundice	Retention less than 70%. No response to two injections of cholecystokinin.
IV	Indeterminate	Retention greater than 70% but less than 90%, and no response to two injections of cholecysto-kinin.

Kelley (32), using the same method as Nordyke and Blahd, confirmed both the sensitivity and reliability of the [131]I- rose bengal test in the diagnosis of hepatocellular dysfunction and biliary obstruction, and found it particularly profitable in documenting the patency of the biliary tract in difficult cases. This was qualified by underscoring the areas where inconclusive results may be obtained as in the obstructive phase of acute hepatitis, and in partial choledochal obstruction due to extrabiliary tree pressure and a "ball valve" common duct stone which are associated with a flow of bile into the gut. Scanning the liver and abdomen serially after radioactive rose bengal administration will obviate some of these difficulties (see Chapter 5).

No distinction between non-jaundiced patients with liver disease and normal individuals could be found by monitoring the head and abdomen according to Garcia and co-workers (33). However, the technique was reported as being eminently suitable for differentiating intrahepatic from extrahepatic jaundice.

Schuman *et al.* (34), employed the same technique and found no clear differentiation between chronic liver disease and acute hepatitis of viral or chlorpromazine etiology. In uncomplicated extrahepatic biliary obstruction, the 20-minute ratios and abdominal tracings simulated those curves found in patients with icterus of mixed etiology and viral hepatitis (6 out of 12 cases). Assuming the abdominal probe did not monitor the excretion of activity by the kidneys and the accumulation in the urinary vesical, which is known to occur in liver disease, these patients presumably had incomplete choledochal obstruction. The authors asserted that a rise in the abdominal count rate within one hour of the injection of [131]I- rose bengal ruled out extrahepatic obstruction.

Taplin and associates (35) contend that the simplest and most accurate method of analyzing the radioactive rose bengal head curves is to measure the time of half disappearance directly from the linear strip chart recording (Fig. 2-4). They also felt that the half disappearance time was superior to the 20-minute retention as an index of polygonal cell integrity in differentiating chronic liver disease from normal, and in observing the stressing effect of bromsulfalein on the removal of [131]I- rose bengal. This contention has theoretical merit, because at 5 minutes only 55

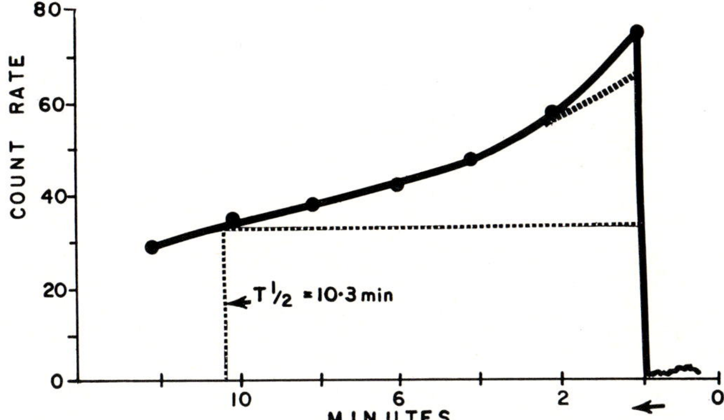

FIGURE 2-4.   Taplin's method of analyzing the [131]I- rose bengal disappearance curve over the head. A linear half-disappearance time is procured by extrapolating the tracing back to zero time to exclude the spike caused by the initial bolus, and reading the time it takes to reach half this count rate.

to 60% of the original blood activity is left in normal individuals, whereas 60 to 100% is present in patients with liver dysfunction. The 5-minute reference point is therefore variable and will tend to increase falsely the retentions in normal subjects to a greater extent than those individuals with liver disease. Thus, a normal retention may be concluded when hepatic disease exists, and an abnormal retention where there is no dysfunction (22). The only difficulty with the half disappearance time calculation is that the curve must be extrapolated to zero by freehand to eliminate the variable bolus effect on the initial rise, and this is subjective.

Taplin et al., obtained a mean half disappearance time of 7.5 minutes in 23 controls, and found the 45-minute bromsulfalein retention more sensitive in detecting liver impairment. However, the concomitant stressing of the [131]I- rose bengal test with bromsulfalein yielded equal or greater sensitivity (35).

Rosenthall conducted a rather extensive study on the use of radioiodinated rose bengal in hepatobiliary disease (36). The method of Blahd and Nordyke (28, 29) was adapted to measure the blood retention, but instead of an abdominal probe to monitor excretion of the radioactive dye into the gut serial scans were obtained. The latter was found to be more reliable, because activity in the bowel can be distinguished from the kidneys and urinary vesical, and the changing distribution within the liver can be appraised (see Chapter 5).

Approximately 25 microcuries [131]I- rose bengal containing 0.1 mg carrier is used when only a clearance study is attempted. If the liver is to be visualized serially, 200 microcuries is administered. A 20-degree divergent collimator is positioned against the side of the head, enclosing the ear, and a continuous recording is produced on a strip chart. The 20-minute retention is procured by taking a ratio of the net 20-minute to the net 5-minute count rate. There is no special preparation of the patient and no attempt is made to incur a fasting state. There is little variation in the results obtained in fasting and postprandial conditions (35).

Normal. The 20-minute retention in 120 normal persons is detailed in Figure 2-5. Normality was assumed when the bili-

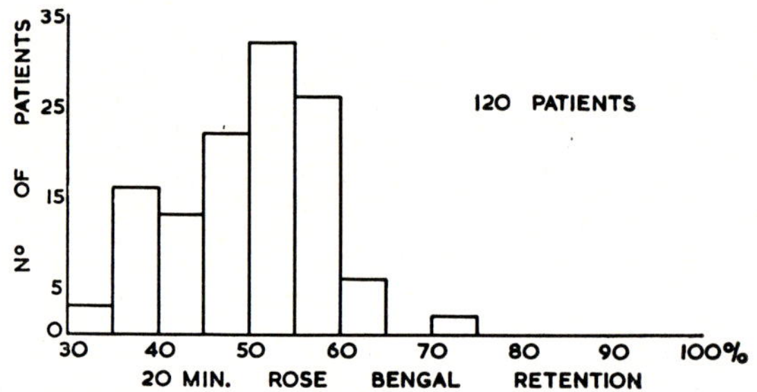

FIGURE 2-5. Histogram of 20-minute [131]I- rose bengal retentions in 120 normal individuals. (Reproduced, courtesy of the *Am. J. Roentgenol., Rad. Therapy & Nuclear Med., 101*:561, 1967.)

rubin, alkaline phosphatase, cephalin flocculation, serum glutamic oxaloacetic transaminase, serum glutamic pyruvic transaminase, bromsulfalein retention and serum proteins were negative. About 95% of the subjects had 20-minute retentions less than 60%, which is higher than the maximum of 50% reported by Nordyke (30). The median was 50%.

Extrahepatic Obstructive Jaundice. Twenty-three out of 24 patients had retentions greater than 60% (Fig. 2-6). A maximum retention of 86% was obtained in 2 patients with complete obstruction of the common duct.

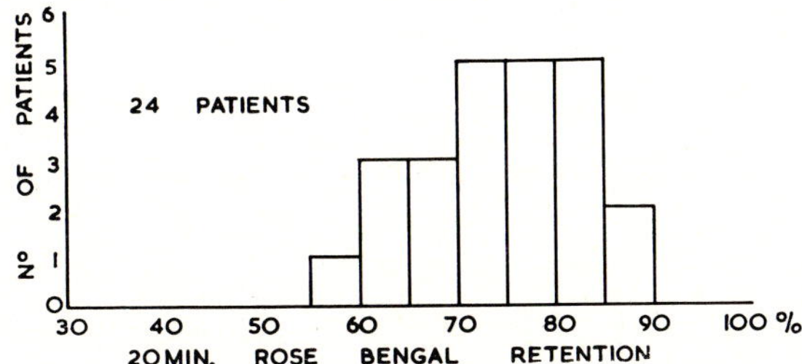

FIGURE 2-6. Histogram of [131]I- rose bengal retentions in 24 patients with extrahepatic obstructive jaundice. (Reproduced, courtesy *Am. J. Roentgenol., Rad. Therapy & Nucl. Med., 101*:561, 1967.)

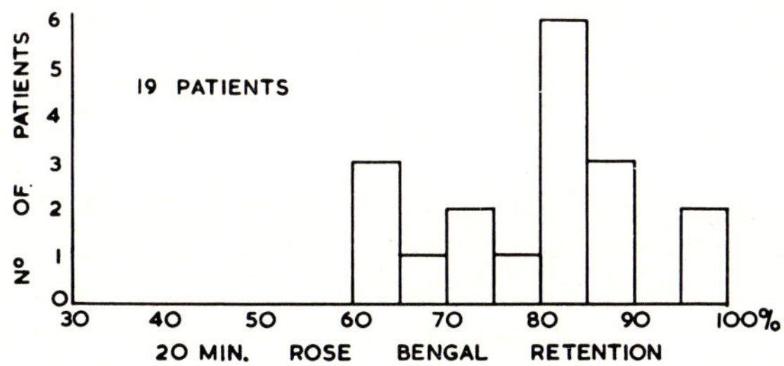

FIGURE 2-7. Histogram of [131]I- rose bengal retentions in 19 patients with acute hepatitis and jaundice. (Reproduced, courtesy *Am. J. Roentgenol., Rad. Therapy & Nucl. Med., 101*:561, 1967.)

Acute Hepatitis and Jaundice. The retentions were similar to the group with extrahepatic obstructive jaundice. All 19 patients had 20-minute retentions exceeding 60% (Fig. 2-7).

Fibrotic Liver Disease Without Jaundice. This group consisted of patients with postnecrotic cirrhosis, nutritional cirrhosis, cardiac cirrhosis, chronic hepatitis, hemochromatosis, biliary cirrhosis, fatty liver with fibrosis, and amyloid disease. All were proved by needle biopsy, laparotomy, or clinically obvious disease. The [131]I- rose bengal retentions varied from 40 to 90%, with a median of 65% (Fig. 2-8). Thirteen out of 49 patients fell into the normal range of 60% or less, which is in partial agreement with other authors who claim that the [131]I- rose bengal test is insensitive to minor liver impairment. A comparative study with bromsulfalein retention was not made.

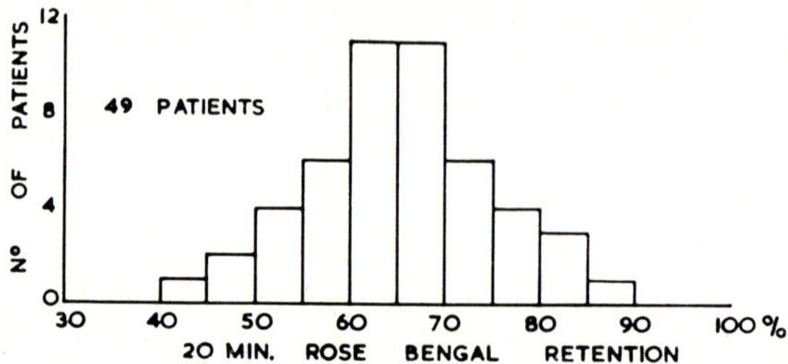

FIGURE 2-8. Histogram of ^{131}I- rose bengal retentions in 49 patients with fibrotic liver disease, but no jaundice. (Reproduced, courtesy *Am. J. Roentgenol., Rad. Therapy & Nucl. Med., 101*:561, 1967.)

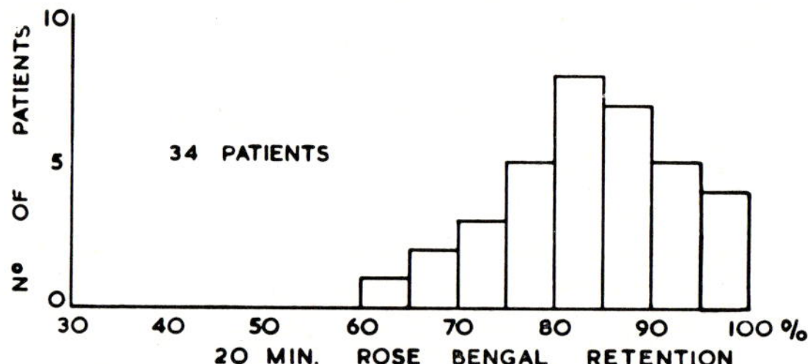

FIGURE 2-9. Histogram of ^{131}I- rose bengal retentions in 34 patients with fibrotic liver disease and jaundice. (Reproduced, courtesy *Am. J. Roentgenol., Rad. Therapy & Nucl. Med., 101*:561, 1967.)

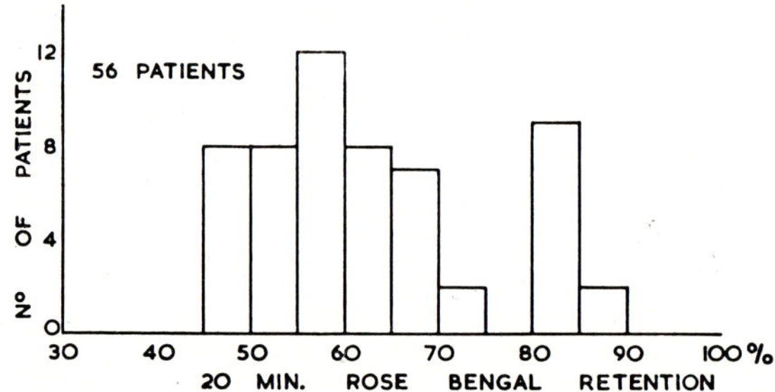

FIGURE 2-10. Histogram of ^{131}I- rose bengal retentions in 56 patients with livers containing primary or metastatic neoplasia. (Reproduced, courtesy *Am. J. Roentgenol., Rad. Therapy, & Nucl. Med., 101*:561, 1967.)

Fibrotic Liver Disease With Jaundice. All 34 patients had retentions greater than 60% (Fig. 2-9).

Liver Containing Tumor. Fifty-six patients were studied who had primary or metastatic neoplasms in the liver. The retentions ranged from 45 to 90%, and were entirely unpredictable (Fig. 2-10).

BIBLIOGRAPHY

1. DELPRAT, G. D., JR.: Studies on liver function: Rose bengal elimination from the blood as influenced by liver injury. *Arch. Int. Med.,* 32:401, 1923.
2. DELPRAT, G. D., JR., EPSTEIN, N. N., AND KERR, W. J.: A new liver function test: The elimination of rose bengal when injected into the circulation of human subjects. *Arch. Int. Med.,* 34:533, 1924.
3. KERR, W. J., DELPRAT, D. G., EPSTEIN, N. N., AND DUNIEVITZ, M.: The rose bengal test for liver function: Studies on the rates of elimination from the circulation in man. *J.A.M.A.,* 85:942, 1925.
4. EPSTEIN, N. N., DELPRAT, G. D., AND KERR, W. J.: The rose bengal test for liver function: Further studies. *J.A.M.A.,* 88:1619, 1927.
5. STOWE, W. P., DELPRAT, G. D., AND WEEKS, A.: The rose bengal test of hepatic function. *J. Lab. and Clin. Med.,* 18:954, 1933.
6. ALTHAUSEN, T. L., BISKIND, G. R., AND KERR, W. T.: The rose bengal test of hepatic function. *J. Lab. and Clin. Med.,* 18:954, 1933.
7. MONROE, L., AND HOPPER, J.: A comparison of the bromsulfalein and rose bengal tests. *J. Lab. and Clin. Med.,* 34:246, 1949.
8. TAPLIN, G. V., MEREDITH, O. M., AND KADE, H.: The radioactive (I^{131} tagged) rose bengal uptake excretion test for liver function using external gamma-ray scintillation counting techniques. *USAEC Report UCLA-319,* University of California at Los Angeles, 1954.
9. TAPLIN, G. V., MEREDITH, O. M., AND KADE, H.: The radioactive (^{131}I tagged) rose bengal uptake excretion test for liver function using external gamma-ray scintillation counting techniques. *J. Lab. and Clin. Med.,* 45:665, 1955.
10. TAPLIN, G. V., MEREDITH, O. M., AND KADE, H.: Development of a radioisotope tracer test for the differential diagnosis of jaundice. *J. Louisiana State Med. Soc.,* 109:255, 1957.
11. ENGLER, T. E., BURROWS, B. A., AND INGELFINGER, F. J.: Quantitative evaluation of hepatic uptake and release of radioactive rose bengal. *Clin. Res. Proc.,* 5:209, 1957.
12. COHN, E. D., ZAGERMAN, J., SKLAROFF, D. M., AND TUMEN, H. J.: The use of radioactive rose bengal as a test in the differential diagnosis of jaundice. *Am. J. Gastroenterology,* 28:621, 1957.
13. BROWN, C. H., AND GLASSER, O.: Radioactive (I^{131}- tagged) rose bengal liver function test. *J. Lab. and Clin. Med.,* 48:454, 1956.
14. LOWENSTEIN, J. M.: Radioactive rose bengal test as a quantitative measure of liver function. *Proc. Soc. Exper. Biol. & Med.,* 93:377, 1956.
15. LOWENSTEIN, J. M.: Quantitative analysis of the radioactive rose bengal test of liver function. *Clin. Res. Proc.,* 5:39, 1957.
16. MOERTEL, C. G., AND OWEN, C. A.: Evaluation of the radioactive (I^{131} tagged) rose bengal liver function test in non-jaundiced patients. *J. Lab. and Clin. Med.,* 52:902, 1958.

17. RICHMAN, A., AND JACOBS, W.: The radioactive (I[131]) rose bengal test of liver function. *J. of the Mt. Sinai Hosp.*, 27:600, 1960.

18. WESTOVER, J. L., GREENFIELD, M. A., AND NORMAN, A.: A clinically useful liver function test using radioactive rose bengal. *J. Lab. and Clin. Med.*, 54:174, 1959.

19. LUM, C. H., MARSHALL, W. J., KOZOLL, D. D., AND MEYER, C. A.: The use of radioactive (I[131]) labelled rose bengal in the study of human liver disease. *Ann. Surg.*, 149:353, 1959.

20. KAWAGUCHI, M., BERK, J. F., AND SOBLE, A. R.: Studies with I[131] labeled rose bengal. Clinical evaluation of a modified technic for differential diagnosis of jaundice. *Am. J. Digest. Dis.*, 7:300, 1962.

21. BERK, J. E., KAWAGUCHI, M., SOBLE, A. R., AND GOLDSTEIN, D. E.: Differential diagnosis of jaundice: Modified I[131]- labeled rose bengal test. *Arch. Int. Med.*, 111:323, 1963.

22. LUSHBAUGH, C. C., KRETCHMAR, A., AND GIBBS, W.: Liver function measured by the blood clearance of rose bengal -I[131]: A review and a model based on compartmental analysis of changes in arm, blood and liver radioactivity. In, *Dynamic Clinical Studies with Radio-isotopes.* Proceedings of a Symposium held at the Oak Ridge Institute of Nuclear Studies, Oct. 21-25, 1963. Edited by R. M. Kniseley, W. N. Tauxe, and E. B. Anderson. Published by U. S. Atomic Energy Commission/Division of Technical Information.

23. COHEN, E. S., GIANSIRACUSA, J. E., AND ALTHAUSEN, T. L.: Studies on bromsulfalein excretion: The simultaneous performance of the bromsulfalein and rose bengal excretion tests in individuals with normal hepatic function. *Gastroenterology*, 25:273, 1953.

24. MENDELOFF, A. I.: Fluorescence of intravenously administered rose bengal appears only in polygonal cells. *Proc. Soc. Exper. Biol. & Med.*, 54:167, 1959.

25. MENA, I., KIVEL, R., MAHONEY, P., MELLINKOFF, S. M., AND BENNETT, L. R.: A method for increasing the sensitivity of the rose bengal I[131] liver function test with the use of bronsulphalein. *J. Lab. and Clin. Med.*, 54:167, 1959.

26. DYRBYE, M. O., AND CHRISTENSEN, L. K.: Clinical value of the radio-active rose bengal liver function test. *Acta Medica Scandinavika*, 167:239, 1960.

27. ACKERMAN, N. B., AND McFEE, A. S.: Malignant obstructive jaundice as detected by levels of rose bengal in the blood after twenty-four hours. *Surgical Forum*, 12:381, 1961.

28. BLAHD, W. H., AND NORDYKE, R. A.: The blood disappearance of radioactive rose bengal. A rapid simple test of liver function. *Clin. Res. Proc.*, 5:40, 1957.

29. NORDYKE, R. A., AND BLAHD, W. A.: Blood disappearance of radio-active rose bengal—Rapid simple test of liver function. *J.A.M.A.*,

30. NORDYKE, R. A.: Surgical vs. non-surgical jaundice. Differentiation by a combination of rose bengal I-131 and standard liver function tests. *J.A.M.A., 194*:949, 1965.

31. NORDYKE, R. A., AND BLAHD, W. H.: The differential diagnosis of biliary tract obstruction with radioactive rose bengal. *J. Lab. Clin. Med., 51*:565, 1958.

32. KELLEY, R. R.: Radioactive rose bengal test—Its use in the diagnosis of liver disease. *Hawaiian Med. J., 24*:362, 1965.

33. GARCIA, A. M., AHMAD, K., WEGST, A. V., AND BEIERWALTES, W. H.: I^{131}- rose bengal test of liver function: A clinical evaluation. *Gastroenterology, 37*:725, 1959.

34. SCHUMAN, B. M., REYNOLDS, W. A., AND EYLER, W. R.: The limitations of the I^{131}- rose bengal liver function test in the differential diagnosis of jaundice. *Gastroenterology, 45*:73, 1963.

35. TAPLIN, G. V., HAYASHI, J., JOHNSON, D. E., AND DORE, E.: Liver blood flow and cellular function in hepatobiliary disease. Tracer studies with radiogold and rose bengal. *J. Nuc. Med., 2*:204, 1961.

36. ROSENTHALL, L.: The application of colloidal radiogold and radio-iodinated rose bengal in hepatobiliary disease. *Am. J. Roentgenol., Rad. Therapy and Nuclear Med., 101*:561, 1967.

Chapter 3

COLLOIDAL RADIOGOLD CLEARANCE AS A PARAMETER OF LIVER PERFUSION IN HEALTH AND HEPATOBILIARY DISEASE

BRADLEY AND CO-WORKERS (1) were the first to describe a clinical procedure for estimating hepatic blood flow, according to the Fick principle, in 1945. It entailed hepatic vein catheterization for repeated blood samplings and a continuous bromsulfalein infusion. This restricted its use to selected patients, and, therefore, was not widely applied. In 1951, Sheppard *et al.* (2), studied the distribution and peripheral blood disappearance of radiogold particles measuring 20 to 100 millimicrons in dogs. Most of the activity lodged in the liver and spleen, and both were equally effective in clearing the particles gram for gram, but the contribution of the spleen was not too significant because of its small size relative to the liver. The exponential feature of particle removal from the peripheral blood led the authors to suggest that this modality might be used to calculate the liver blood flow.

Assuming a mono-exponential removal of colloidal material, the resultant curve of peripheral activity versus time can be expressed as $A = A_o e^{-kt}$, where Ao is the amount of radioactivity injected, A is radioactivity still in circulation at time t, and K is the disappearance rate constant. K may be considered as the fraction of the total amount of activity administered which is removed per minute by the liver, assuming that the liver is the only site of deposition, and it is completely removed with each passage through the organ. If B is the total body blood volume, Q is the combined hepatic artery and portal vein blood flows, and T½ is the half disappearance time of the particles from the circulation, then

$$Q = KB = \frac{0.69B}{T\frac{1}{2}}$$

When the particles are not completely removed by the liver, the observed T½ is falsely elevated and a minimum estimated hepatic blood flow is calculated from the above equation.

The corrected relationship is:

$$Q = \frac{KB}{E} = \frac{0.69B}{E\ T\frac{1}{2}}$$

where E is the fraction of the particles extracted by the liver from a single passage through the organ.

Dobson and Jones (3) conducted an intensive investigation on the use of colloidal chromic phosphate labelled with radiophosphorous for the measurement of hepatic perfusion. The method consisted of an intravenous injection of the test agent followed by serial blood sample assays to plot its disappearance from the peripheral circulation as a function of time. At least two exponential components were derived from the resultant curve. Liver blood flow was calculated from the half disappearance time of the fast component only. This was based on the assumption that the slower components were caused by the small particles of the chromic phosphate preparation spectrum which were not phagocytosed by the Kupffer cells. Rankin and associates (4) recovered 80% of the chromic phosphate from the liver and spleen following ante mortem administration in three normal livers at autopsy, but only from 26 to 56% in five patients with cirrhosis. The bone marrow was the major alternative site of colloidal deposition. This reduction in extraction efficiency is due to intrahepatic bypassing of the Kupffer cells lining the sinusoidal pathway, and it is variable in degree. If a normal value of E [about 0.82 (5)] is used in the liver blood flow equation, Q will be grossly underestimated in cirrhosis. Thus, Rankin *et al.*, feel their findings invalidate the method using colloidal chromic phosphate for the absolute measurement of total hepatic blood flow in the presence of impaired liver function, although adequate otherwise.

[131]I heat denatured albumin was introduced by Halpern *et al.* (6, 7), because a smaller spectrum of particle size and a larger fraction of clearance, E, could be obtained for liver blood flow measurements. Shaldon *et al.* (8), extended their work, and found the method valid in normal subjects. It underestimated liver blood flow in cirrhotics by the amount of blood shunted through the intrahepatic portal-hepatic venous anastomoses, which are not lined by Kupffer cells.

Vetter and co-workers (9) introduced colloidal [198]Au as an agent to measure hepatic blood flow. They felt that the gamma emitting properties of radiogold, which permits external monitoring of the peripheral circulation, is more desirable than the multiple venapunctures necessitated by chromic phosphate. Furthermore, the laborious preparation of chromic phosphate of suitable particle size is obviated. The average size of the gold particles employed in their investigation was 25 millimicrons. A semi-logarithmic plot of the tracing obtained over the calves yielded a multi-exponential disappearance curve. Only the fast component was used to calculate liver blood flow, because the slower components were thought to represent a more gradual extrasplanchnic removal of the smaller particles which were not phagocytosed by the Kupffer cells (10). In three normal individuals, the fraction of clearance, E, was determined at 0.80. This figure has come under some criticism because commercial preparations vary in their particle size spectrum, and the efficiency of Kupffer cell trapping varies with the size (11). The colloidal preparations all suffer from the same shortcomings in liver disease associated with intrahepatic circulatory shunting, and will underestimate total liver blood flow unless accompanied by catheter studies to measure E in each case, but this defeats the simplicity of the original intent.

Splenic injection of [131]I- human serum albumin in patients with cirrhosis demonstrated a diversion of 22 to 81% of the portal blood to the collateral vessels (12). A large spleen is capable of extracting a significant number of particles, and in the presence of a large collateral bypass it will tend to reduce the half disappearance time, T½, or reciprocally increase the disappearance rate constant, K. It was demonstrated that K is larger in patients with collaterals than in patients without them, and this will give a higher estimated liver blood flow than exists. To circumvent this, it is suggested that the hepatic uptake of radiogold should be monitored rather than blood clearance (12). External hepatic monitoring of the uptake of [131]I- denatured albumin is also preferred by Torrance and Gowenlock (5), because the curves are mono-exponential as opposed to multi-exponential when derived over the head. Baptista and Carvalho (13) are partial to monitoring the liver uptake of radiogold to determine blood flow, because smaller doses can be employed and better counting statistics are obtained.

A comparative study of bromsulfalein and colloidal [198]Au methods of hepatic blood flow was made by Vetter *et al.* (14), in fifteen normal persons. The results of colloidal radiogold were 15.6% lower. This was attributed to incomplete mixing, small fractions of radiogold detention in the bone marrow, adrenals and kidneys, and an 18% escape of large and medium sized particles on each passage through the liver. At autopsy, 90 to 95% of the radiogold was recovered in the liver and spleen (15).

Above a critical quantity of colloidal material, the disappearance rate constant, K, will decrease. At this point, the K is no longer blood flow limited, but an index of phagocytosis of the total mass of cells for the given quantity of administered colloid (16). The quantity of colloidal gold should be kept below 250 micrograms to avoid saturation (9).

Portal vein ligated rats show that the hepatic artery is capable of supplying from 30 to 40% of the liver blood flow with chromic phosphate as the test agent (3). Anaesthetized patients exhibited a lower blood flow than conscious patients (17), and epinephrine greatly depresses the perfusion (3).

K values culled from the literature are tabulated below:

Authors	Test Agent	K (Normal)	K (Cirrhosis)
Vetter *et al.* (9)	[198]Au	0.269*	0.095
		0.242†	
Krook (18)	[198]Au	0.158	0.092
Baptista and Carvalho (13)	[198]Au	0.296	
Riddel *et al.* (19)	[198]Au	0.169	
Burkle and Gliedman (20)	[198]Au	0.196	

Fauvert (21)	^{198}Au	0.166	
	Bromsulfalein	0.145	
Antognetti *et al.* (22)	^{198}Au	0.220	0.075
Nardi *et al.* (23)	Chromic PO$_4$	0.303*	
		0.350†	
Torrance and Gowenlock (5)	Chromic PO$_4$	0.238	
Halpern (16)	^{131}I denatured albumin	0.318*	0.175
		0.350†	
Shaldon *et al.* (8)	^{131}I denatured albumin	0.339	0.288

---

* Male
† Female

Despite the objections to using radioactive colloidal material for measuring absolute total blood flow in liver, the shape of the disappearance curve does reflect qualitatively the hepatic perfusion, particularly the functional or sinusoidal flow which is known to be reduced in cirrhosis. By a corrosive castive technique Carter *et al.* (24), recorded volumetric changes in the hepatic vasculature of eight normal and eight cirrhotic livers at necropsy. The vascular volume averaged 213 grams in normal livers and 137 grams in cirrhotic livers. This 36% decrease in vascular volume compared to a 10% loss in total liver weight indicated a relatively greater vascular than parenchymal loss in cirrhotics. The inflow tract volume in the normal liver, hepatic artery plus portal vein, was 112 grams, and the outflow tract, hepatic vein, was 101 grams. In cirrhosis, the inflow tract was 89 grams and the outflow tract 49 grams; the hepatic venous system showing a preponderently greater reduction.

Taplin *et al.* (25) used the time of half-disappearance of the colloidal ^{198}Au as an index of functional perfusion, and it was measured directly from the rectilinear tracing obtained over the head by extrapolating the curve back to zero freehand to exclude the initial spike due to the bolus effect. The linear half-times derived by this method were almost identical to the more time consuming exponential analysis in normal subjects. On the other hand, in proved cirrhotics with portal hypertension the linear half-time values were proportionately greater than the values calculated by the exponential method, thus the latter tends to minimize the estimated impairment of liver blood flow. The following half-disappearance times, T½, are adapted from the data published by Taplin *et al.* (25, 26).

Diagnosis	Number of Patients	Mean T½ (minutes)	Range of T½ (minutes)
Normal	28	4.5	2.7 — 5.3
Alcoholism, chronic	15	5.0	3.3 — 6.8
Cirrhosis, compensated	26	8.5	4.1 — 15.0
Cirrhosis, decompensated	46	15.4	5.0 — 29.0
Cirrhosis, porto-caval shunt	11	18.2	11.2 — 30+
Hepatitis, acute	41	4.5	2.7 — 6.3
Obstructive jaundice	23	4.5	2.7 — 6.1

It is stressed that the half-disappearance time (T½) and the disappearance rate constant (K) are only indices of effective blood flow to the liver and spleen, but they provide practical information in evaluating cirrhotics and serially studying other hepatobiliary dysfunctions (26).

To evaluate hepatocellular dysfunction relative to liver blood flow, a ratio of the ^{131}I- rose bengal to the colloidal ^{198}Au half-disappearance times (26) or clearances (27) may give some qualitative information. The following are the values reported by Taplin *et al.* (26).

Diagnosis	Number of Patients	$\dfrac{^{131}I\text{- Rose Bengal, }T½}{Colloidal\ ^{198}Au,\ T½}$
Controls	28	1.8 ± 0.2
Alcoholism, chronic	15	2.1 ± 0.3
Cirrhosis, compensated	26	2.0 ± 0.5
Cirrhosis, decompensated	46	2.1 ± 1.1
Hepatitis, acute	41	6.0 ± 3.4
Obstructive jaundice	23	5.5 ± 2.2

The normal ^{131}I- rose bengal to colloidal ^{198}Au ratio is approximately 2. A similar value is obtained in cirrhosis and chronic hepatitis, unless there is a superimposed hepatocellular dysfunction, in which case the ratio exceeds 2 by the degree of polygonal cell impairment.

Rosenthall (29) also carried out a correlative assessment of the peripheral disappearance of radiogold by external monitoring of the head in a variety of hepatobiliary dysfunctions. However, instead of measuring a linear half-disappearance time, a ratio of the net 4.5 minute count rate to the net 1.5 minute count rate was obtained, or a "4.5 minute ^{198}Au retention" (Fig. 3-1). This interval was used because of the short existence of the larger particles in the vasculature, and the minute or so it takes the

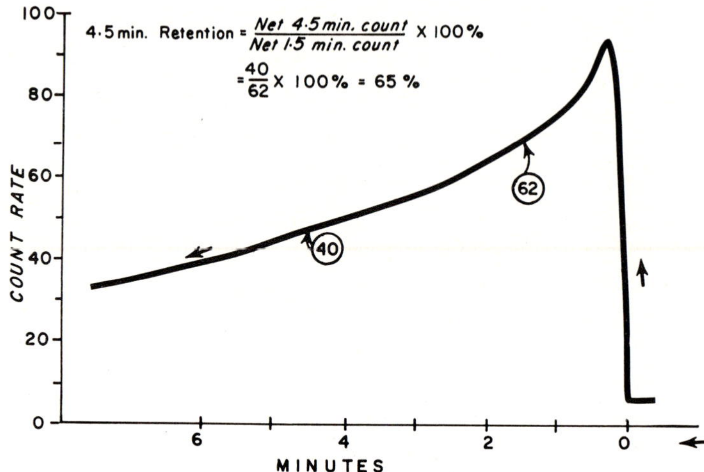

FIGURE 3-1.   A radiogold disappearance curve obtained over the head with
an external scintillation detector in a normal individual. The 4.5-minute
[198]Au retention is the ratio of the net 4.5-minute count rate to the net
1.5-minute count rate.

tracing to settle after the initial bolus in some patients. A dose
of approximately 25 microcuries [198]Au was employed if only a
retention curve was desired, but when a liver scan was to follow
200 microcuries was administered.

Figure 3-2 is the histogram obtained in 116 patients with
normal liver function tests, which included bilirubin, alkaline

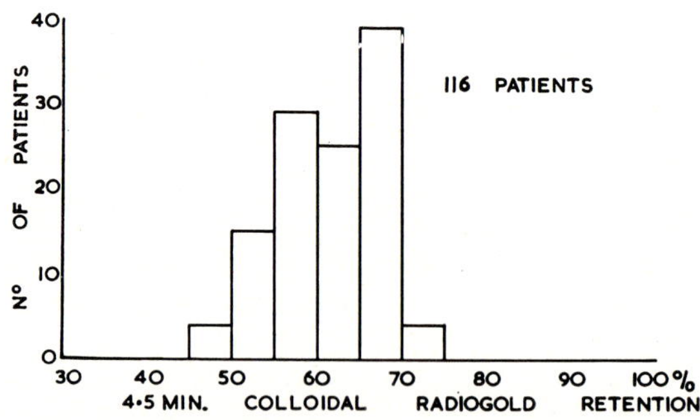

FIGURE 3-2.   Histogram of 4.5-minute [198]Au retentions in 116 normal
subjects. (Reproduced, courtesy of the *American Journal of Roentgenology,
Rad. Therapy & Nucl. Med., 101*:561, 1967.

phosphatase, cephalin flocculation, serum glutamic oxaloacetic transaminase (SGOT), serum glutamic pyruvic transaminase (SGPT), and bromsulfalein. Approximately 95% of the controls had a 4.5-minute [198]Au retention less than 70%. The median was 50%.

The histogram of 54 patients with fibrotic liver disease, but no jaundice or ascites, is presented in Figure 3-3. These included proved cases of postnecrotic cirrhosis, nutritional cirrhosis, cardiac cirrhosis, chronic hepatitis, hemochromatosis, biliary cirrhosis, fatty liver with fibrosis, and amyloid disease. The 4.5-minute [198]Au retentions varied from 50 to 100%. All 12 patients with gold retentions less than 70% had large fatty livers with some fibrosis on histological examination of the needle biopsy specimen. Many of them had a history of high alcohol intake and the observed findings most likely represented early nutritional

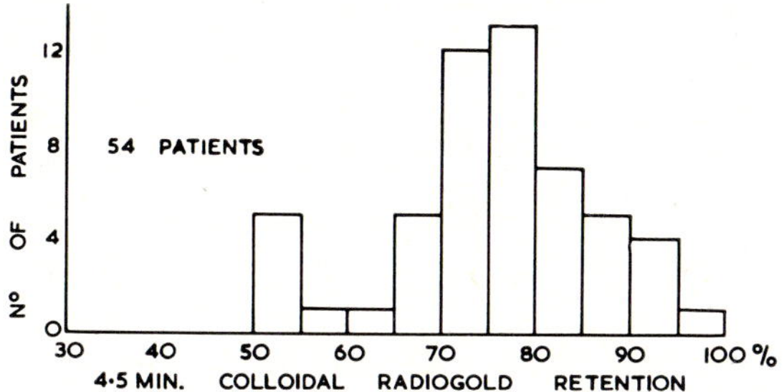

FIGURE 3-3.   Histogram of 4.5-minute [198]Au retentions in 54 patients with fibrotic liver disease, but no icterus or ascites.

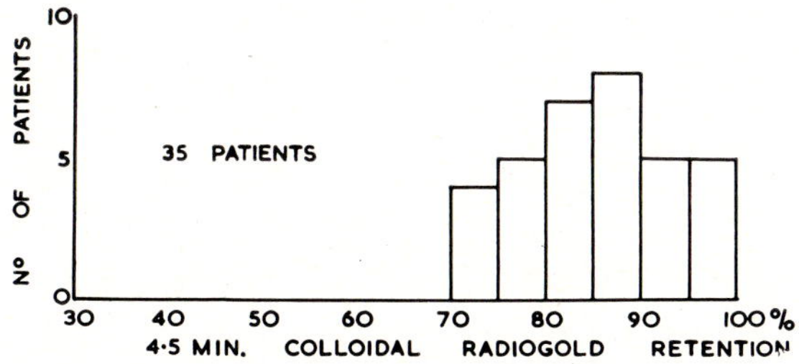

FIGURE 3-4.   Histogram of 4.5-minute [198]Au retentions in 35 patients with fibrotic liver disease and jaundice, with or without ascites.

cirrhosis, but too early in its genesis to be detected by the radiogold function study.

All 35 patients with fibrotic liver disease and jaundice, with or without ascites, had 4.5 minute [198]Au retentions exceeding 70% (Fig. 3-4).

Of the 19 patients with acute hepatitis and jaundice, 16 had 4.5-minute retentions less than 70%, one had a retention of 72% and 2 exceeded 80% (Fig. 3-5). The latter two had acute yellow atrophy with retentions below 70% earlier in the course of the

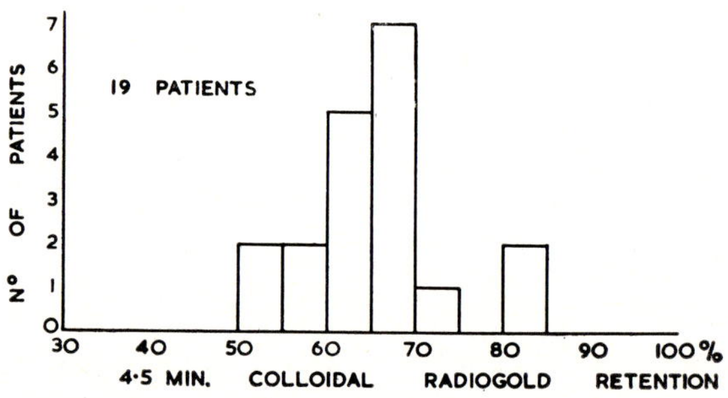

Figure 3-5.   Histogram of 4.5 minute [198]Au retentions in 19 patients with acute hepatitis and jaundice.

illness. Thus, a persistence or deepening of the icterus and a rising 4.5-minute [198]Au retention portends deterioration. A reduction in liver size can accompany this change. Otherwise, a retention greater than 70% in a patient who is jaundiced, with or without ascites, indicates an underlying chronic process.

Twenty-seven out of 28 patients with obstructive jaundice had 4.5-minute retentions less than 70% (Figure 3-6). Seven cases of intrahepatic cholestasis, not included in this series, also had retentions less than 70%.

Patients in congestive heart failure generally had radiogold retentions in the upper limits of normal; that is, between 60 and 70%. A few with retentions greater than 70% reverted to normal following digitalization. The radiogold retentions are not a satisfactory substitute for cardiac output measurements.

Livers involved with neoplasm gave unpredictable results (Fig. 3-7). The retentions varied from 50 to 95%. There was a

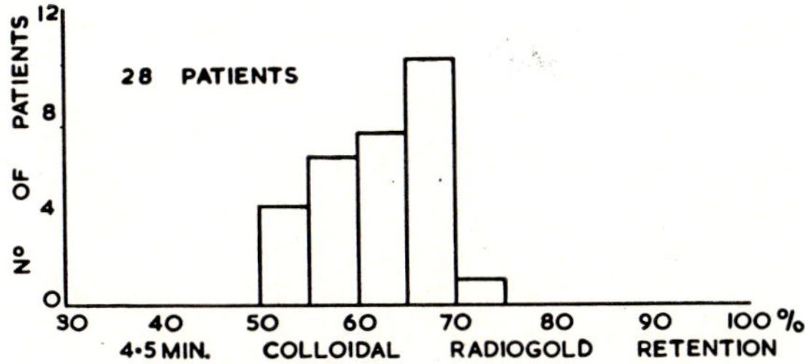

FIGURE 3-6.   Histogram of 4.5-minute [198]Au retentions in 28 patients with extrahepatic obstructive jaundice.

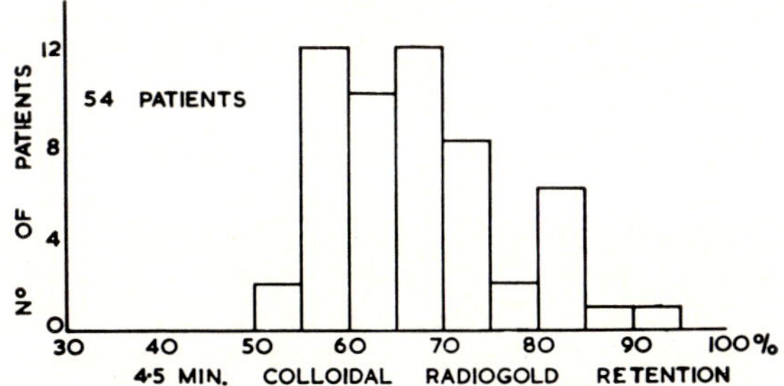

FIGURE 3-7.   Histogram of 4.5-minute [198]Au retentions in 54 patients with primary and secondary tumors of the liver.

tendency for a higher retention with a greater degree of tumor replacement. This is in keeping with the findings reported following hepatic vein catheterization, which showed a greatly reduced particle extraction efficiency in blood draining the tumor bed (29). These studies also demonstrated an increased total hepatic blood flow. A striking example of hepatic artery—hepatic vein shunting of macroaggregates of radioiodinated albumin (MARIA) measuring between 10 and 30 microns, in a patient with extensive liver deposits of a testicular choriocarcinoma, is shown in Fig. 3-8. The MARIA was injected into the celiac axis, and the concentration in the lung, the shunted moiety, approximates the liver concentration. This method cannot be used to measure the fraction of the total hepatic blood flow bypassing the sinusoids, because tumor vessels smaller than 10 microns in diameter will trap the MARIA.

The mean 20-minute [131]I- rose bengal ([131]IRB) and the 4.5-

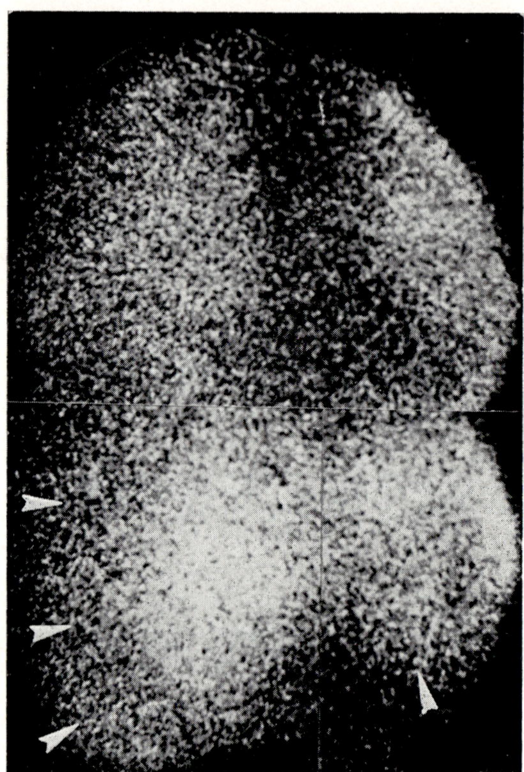

FIGURE 3-8.   Composite lung and liver scan obtained following celiac axis injection of [131]I- macroaggregates of albumin in a patients with liver metastases from a testicular choriocarcinoma. The concentration of particles in the lungs was due to hepatic artery-venous shunting through the tumor bed. (Arrows indicate areas of liver replacement by tumor.)

minute [198]Au retentions, and their ratios, for the various hepatobiliary afflictions discussed are as follows:

Diagnosis	Mean 4.5 min. [198]Au (%)	Mean 20 min. [131]IRB (%)	20 min. [131]IRB / 4.5 min. [198]Au
Normal	60	50	0.83
Hepatitis, acute	60	80	1.33
Extrahepatic obstructive jaundice	60	75	1.25
Fibrotic liver disease without jaundice	75	65	0.86
Fibrotic liver disease with jaundice	85	85	1.00
Tumor	65	60	0.92

It would appear from the ratios that a value of one or greater is indicative of a superimposed polygonal cell failure if the

4.5-minute radiogold retention is elevated. When the ratios are less than one, the elevated 20-minute [131]I- rose bengal retention may be due to reduced hepatic perfusion primarily.

BIBLIOGRAPHY

1. Bradley, S. E., Ingelfinger, F. J., Bradley, G. P., and Curry, J. J.: Estimation of the hepatic blood flow in man. *J. Clin. Investigation,* *94*:890, 1945.
2. Sheppard, C. W., Jordan, G., and Hahn, P. H.: Disappearance of isotopically labelled gold colloids from the circulation of the dog. *Am. J. Physiology, 164*:345, 1951.
3. Dobson, E. L., and Jones, E. L.: The behaviour of intravenously injected particulate material: Its rate of disappearance from the blood stream as a measure of liver blood flow. *Acta Med. Scand., Suppl., 273*, 1952.
4. Rankin, R. G., Playoust, M. R., and Beal, R. W.: Significance of alterations in extraction and distribution of colloidal chromic phosphate in patients with liver disease. *J. Lab. & Clin. Med.,* 58:920, 1961.
5. Torrance, H. B., and Gowenlock, A. H.: Radioactive colloidal clearance techniques to measure liver blood flow in man. *Clin. Science,* 22:413, 1962.
6. Halpern, B. N., Biozzi, G., Benacerrof, B., Stiffel, C., and Hillenmand, B.: Cinétique de la Phagocytose d'une Sérum-albumine Humaine Spécialement Traitée et Radiomarquée, et son Application à l'étude de la Circulation Hépatique Chez l'homme. *C. R. Soc. Biol. (Paris), 150*:1307, 1956.
7. Benacerraf, B., Biozzi, G., Halpern, B. N., Stiffel, C., and Mouton, D.: Phagocytosis of heat denatured serum albumin labelled with ^{131}I and its use as a means of investigating liver blood flow. *Brit. J. Exp. Path., 38*:35, 1956.
8. Shaldon, S., Chiandussi, L., Guevara, L., Caesar, J., and Sherlock, S.: The estimation of hepatic blood flow and intrahepatic shunted blood flow by colloidal heat-denatured human serum albumin labeled with I[131]. *J. Clin. Invest., 40*:1346, 1961.
9. Vetter, H., Falkner, R., and Neumayr, A.: The disappearance of colloid Radiogold from the circulation and its application to the estimation of liver blood flow in normal and cirrhotic subjects. *J. Clin. Invest., 33*:1594, 1954.
10. Zilversmit, D. D., Boyd, G. A., and Brucer, M.: The effect of particle size on blood clearance and tissue distribution of radioactive gold colloid. *J. Lab. & Clin. Med., 40*:255, 1952.
11. Playoust, M. R., McRae, J., and Boden, R. W.: Inefficient hepatic

extraction of colloidal gold: Resulting inaccuracies in determination of hepatic blood flow. *J. Lab. & Clin. Med.,* 54:728, 1959.

12. MOUSA, A. H., EL-GAREM, A., EL-ROOBY, A., SAIF, E., AND EL-ABDINE, A. Z.: Evaluation of the BSP and radiogold clearance techniques in estimating hepatic flow in hepatosplenic bilharziasis. *J. Egypt. Med. Assoc.,* 49:33, 1966.

13. BAPTISTA, A. M., AND CARVALHO, J. S.: Study of the liver blood flow using gamma-emitting radionuclides. *Proceedings of the Second International Conference on the Peaceful Uses of Atomic Energy,* 26:157, 1958.

14. VETTER, H., GRABNER, G., HOFER, R., NEUMAYR, A., AND PARKER, O.:

14. VETTER, H., GRABNER, G., HOFER, R., NEUMAYR, A., AND PARZER, O.: Comparison of liver blood flow values estimated by the bromsulphalein and by the radiogold method. *J. Clin. Invest.,* 35:825, 1956.

15. FELLINGER, K., AND VETTER, H.: Radiogold-Therapie der Leukamischen Erkrankungen Strahlenthen, 33:175, 1955.

16. HALPERN, B.: Estimation of the hepatic circulation without catheterization. *Triangle, The Sandoz J. of Med. Science,* 8:117, 1967.

17. TORRANCE, H. P.: The application of an external scintillation counter technique to investigate various aspects of the splanchnic circulation in man. *Rev. Int. Hépat.,* 16:1011, 1966.

18. KROOK, H.: Circulatory studies in liver cirrhosis. *Acta Med. Scand.,* Suppl. *318,* 1956.

19. RIDDEL, A. G., GRIFFITHS, D. D., MCALLISTER, J. M., AND OSBORN, S. B.: The measurement of liver blood flow with colloidal radiogold (Au^{198}). *Clin. Science,* 16:315, 1957.

20. BURKLE, J. S., AND GLIEDMAN, M. L.: External recording method for estimating hepatic blood flow with the use of radiogold. *Gastroenterology,* 36:112, 1959.

21. FAUVERT, R. E.: The concept of hepatic clearance. *Gastroenterology,* 37:603, 1959.

22. ANTOGNETTI, L., FERRINI, O., AND BESTAGNO, M.: Aspetti Applicativi dei Radioisotopi Nella Semeiologica Funzionale del Fegato e dell'aparato. *Gastroenterico Minerva Nuclear,* 4:37, 1960.

23. NARDI, G. L., PLAZZI, H. M., AND LEVY, M. L.: Liver blood flow in man: Studies utilizing radioactive colloid. *Gastroenterology,* 37:295, 1959.

24. CARTER, J. H., WELCH, C. S., AND BARRON, R. E.: Changes in the hepatic blood vessels in cirrhosis of the liver. *Surg., Gynec. and Obstet.,* 113:133, 1961.

25. TAPLIN, G. V., HAYASHI, J., JOHNSON, D. E., AND DORE, E.: Liver blood flow and cellular function in hepatobiliary disease. Tracer studies with radiogold and rose bengal. *J. Nuclear Med.,* 2:204, 1961.

26. TAPLIN, G. V., DORE, E. K., AND JOHNSON, D. E.: Hepatic blood flow

and reticulo-endothelial system studies with radiocolloids. In, *Dynamic Clinical Studies with Radioisotopes.* Edited by R. M. Kniseley, W. Newton Tauxe and E. B. Anderson; Published by U. S. Atomic Energy Commission/Division of Technical Information; 1964, pp. 285.

27. KOCH-WESER, D.: The ratio of colloidal gold-rose bengal clearance as a differential measurement of impaired hepatic blood flow and function. *Strahlentherapie* (Suppl. 5, Strahlenbehandlung), 53:378, 1963.

28. ROSENTHALL, LEONARD: The application of colloidal radiogold and radioiodinated rose bengal in hepatobiliary disease. *Am. J. Roentgenol., Rad. Therapy, & Nuclear Med., 101*:561, 1967.

29. WARTNABY, K. M., BOUCHIER, I. A. D., POPE, C. E., AND SHERLOCK, S.: Hepatic blood flow in patients with tumors of the liver. *Gastroenterology, 44*:733, 1963.

Chapter 4

IMAGING THE LIVER

A TECHNIQUE FOR detecting hepatic neoplasms was described in 1953 by Stirrett, Yuhl and Libby (1). It consisted of an intravenous injection of 300 microcuries of [131]I- human serum albumin, and 24 hours later 42 points were selected over the liver and adjacent areas, and counted with an external detector. The metastatic deposits purportedly exhibited the highest count rates by virtue of their increased vascularity. A 96% accuracy was claimed in 56 selected patients. MacEwan (2), on the other hand, administered [131]I- human serum albumin to four patients shortly before death, and at autopsy could find no selective concentration of radioactive material by the liver tissue or hepatic metastases.

The earliest article on liver mapping with an automatic rectilinear scanner appeared in 1954 (3). Colloidal radiogold was the test agent, and the detector head contained a simple straight bore collimator of three-eighths inch diameter. Since then, focusing collimators were introduced, scintillation crystals were made larger, and stationary-type devices such as the Ter-Pogossian image intensifier (4), the gamma-ray scintillation camera (5), and the autofluoroscope (6) were made commercially available. Most of this equipment can be linked to tape recording and playback systems, television monitoring and ciné, and ultimately to data-processing devices or computers. Despite this array of sophisticated options, the liver lesion detection frequency has not improved commensurately.

A number of gamma emitting radiopharmaceuticals can be employed in liver scanning. These are divided into particulate suspensions which are phagocytosed by the Kupffer cells, and those agents which are concentrated by the parenchymal cells. The former group includes colloidal radiogold (^{198}Au or ^{199}Au), ^{131}I denatured protein (7), technetium-99^{m} thiocyanate in fat emulsion (concentrated by the polygonal cell as well) (8), technetium-99^{m} sulfide colloid (9, 10) and indium-113^{m} colloid (11). Radioactive rose bengal is essentially the only popular radiopharmaceutical in the "parenchymal cell" category, but selenium-75 labelled methionine, zinc-69^{m} chloride (12) and copper-64 can be used.

The following is the absorbed dose for some of these test agents:

Test Agent	Amount Administered		Liver Absorbed Dose in Rads
Colloidal Au-198	150	microcuries	5
Tc-99^{m} sulfide colloid	3	millicuries	0.9
I-131 denatured albumin	150	microcuries	0.09
Indium-113^{m} colloid	3	millicuries	1.65
I-131 rose bengal	150	microcuries	2
Zn-69^{m} chloride	150	microcuries	1

RESOLUTION OF SPACE-OCCUPYING DISEASE

Any lesion which will displace or replace the liver substance, and is large enough to be resolved by the scanning apparatus, will be seen as an area of reduced or absent radioactivity (Fig. 4-1). The minimum size of a lesion which can be detected varies from report to report. Liver phantom studies using ^{131}I and ^{198}Au have shown that spherical lesions as small as 2 cm diameter can be detected (13), and in another communication it is stated that a 2.5 cm diameter defect on the surface of the liver can always be detected, but a 1.7 cm diameter defect is not resolvable (14). A comparison of patients' scans with the surgical findings places the lower limit of detection at 2 cm diameter (15, 16). A similar investigation indicated a lower limit of 1.5 cm diameter in the left lobe and the dome surface of the liver, but stressed that lesions of 2 to 3 cm may not be observed when they are deep in the right lobe (17).

A liver phantom study consisting of an intercomparison of

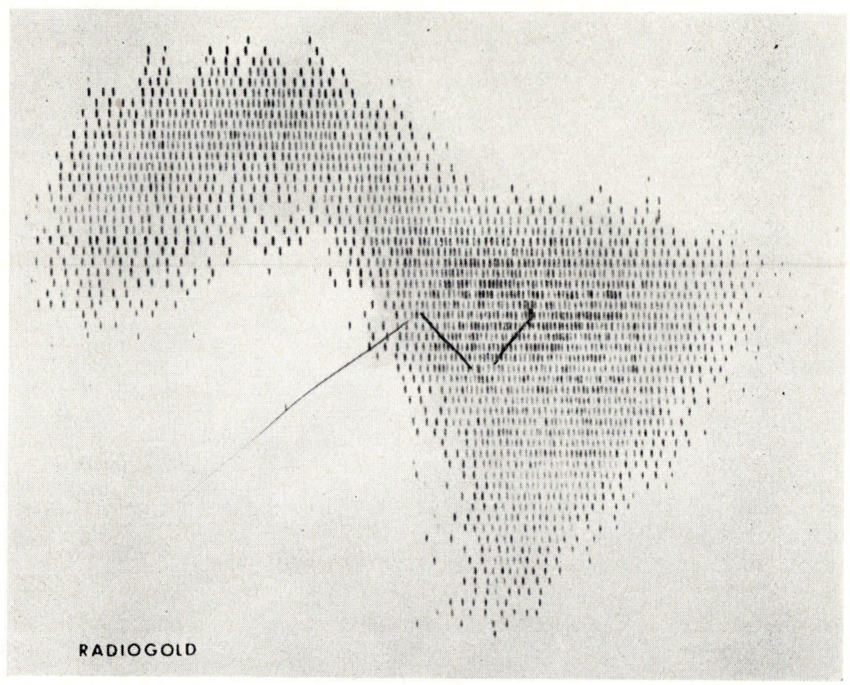

FIGURE 4-1A.   A colloidal ^{198}Au scan of the liver showing a large hepatoma replacing most of the right lobe.

^{99m}Tc, ^{197}Hg, ^{198}Au and ^{131}I for filling defects of various sizes was initiated by Loken and Gerding (18). They found that the smallest detectable surface lesion with ^{99m}Tc and ^{197}Hg was 1.25 cm in diameter. The corresponding values for ^{131}I and ^{198}Au were 1.5 cm and 1.75 cm., respectively. At 8 cm depth a 2.5 cm diameter lesion was barely perceptible with ^{99m}Tc, but the minimum diameter for ^{197}Hg, and ^{198}Au was larger at 3.25 cm. ^{131}I was somewhat better, being 3.25 cm at 9 cm depth.

THE VALUE OF COMBINED FRONTAL AND LATERAL LIVER SCANS

Normal respiration, and overlying ribs and soft tissue structures further reduce the resolution obtained with the liver phantom. In routine practice, a deep-seated lesion measuring 4-5 cm in diameter in the right lobe, and 2-3 cm in the left lobe,

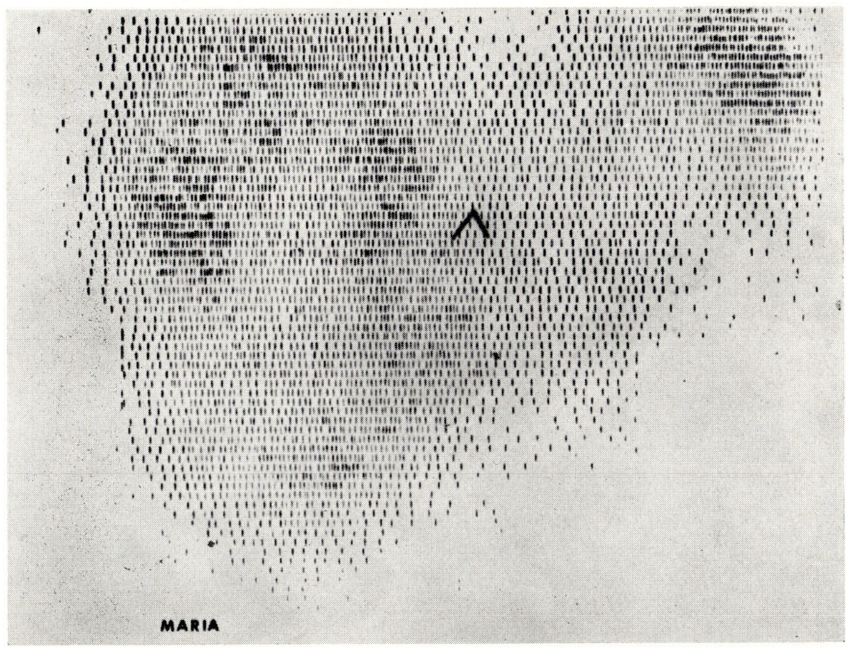

FIGURE 4-1B. Same patient following a celiac axis injection of macro-aggregates of radioiodinated albumin (MARIA), which ranged from 10 to 30 microns in size. The abundant vasculature of the hepatoma trapped the MARIA, but the neoplasm will not concentrate the usual test agents like rose bengal and colloidal gold.

may escape detection. Anterior, posterior, and lateral scans of the liver have been advocated to minimize the depth factor. Czerniak analyzed 65 cases of hepatic echinococcosis, and found more information was gained in 73% of the cases when the lateral view was combined with the conventional frontal examination (19). In a small series of 34 consecutive proved abnormal livers, Rosenthall and Usher obtained the following results with colloidal radiogold as the test agent (20):

Lesion	Number of Patients	%
Seen on lateral scan only	7	20
Frontal scan suspicious, but lateral scan definitely abnormal	10	30
Seen on both frontal and lateral scans	14	41
Seen on frontal scan only	3	9

Inasmuch as the lateral projection was fully helpful in making a diagnosis in 50% of the cases it should be included with the frontal scan in the routine liver study.

Figure 4-2 is a frontal and right lateral colloidal [198]Au scan

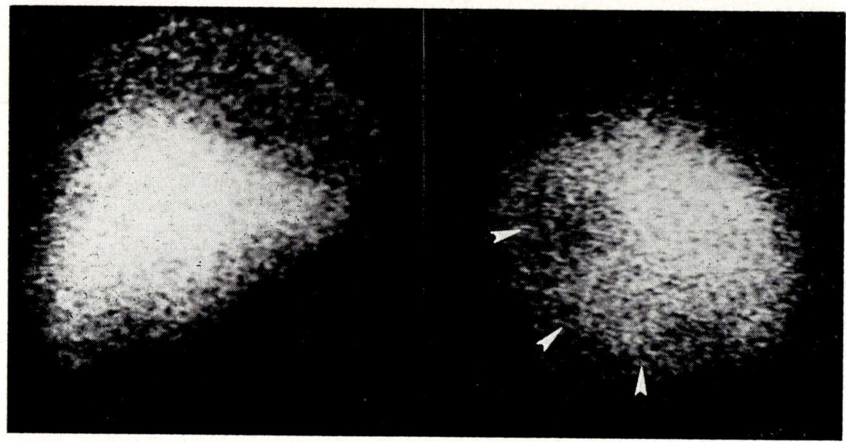

FIGURE 4-2. Frontal (*left*) and lateral (*right*) radiogold liver scans of a patient with known metastatic carcinoma of the colon. The frontal projection is normal, but the lateral view depicts considerable replacement of the posterior section of the right lobe (*arrows*).

of the liver in a patient known to have carcinoma of the colon. The frontal projection shows no evidence of metastatic disease, but the lateral scan clearly portrays replacement of a large posterior segment of the right lobe.

A similar example of a normal frontal, but abnormal lateral scan is illustrated in Figure 4-3. The patient had known metastatic deposits from a gastric carcinoma, and most of the posterior half of the right lobe was destroyed.

The frontal scan may be questionable, and the lateral view definitive. Figure 4-4, a case in point, represents the frontal and lateral views of the liver in a patient with breast carcinomatosis. The frontal scan showed some hypoactivity in the superior half of the left lobe, and the spleen contained more activity than normally found, the latter indicating portal hypertension and/or intrahepatic shunting. There was almost complete destruction of the posterior half of the right lobe when seen from the side.

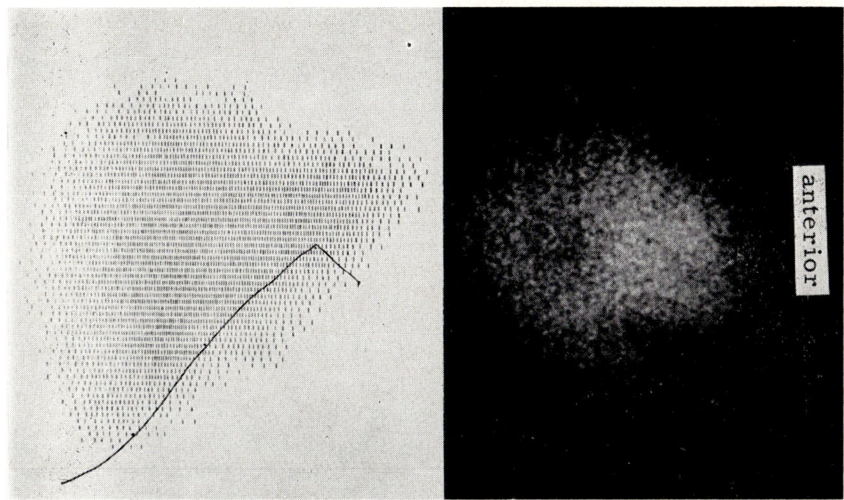

FIGURE 4-3. Frontal (*left*) and lateral (*right*) colloidal ^{198}Au liver scans of a patient with a gastric carcinoma destroying most of the right lobe, but seen only in the right lateral projection. (Reproduced, courtesy of the *Journal of the Canadian Association of Radiologists, 17*:151, 1966.)

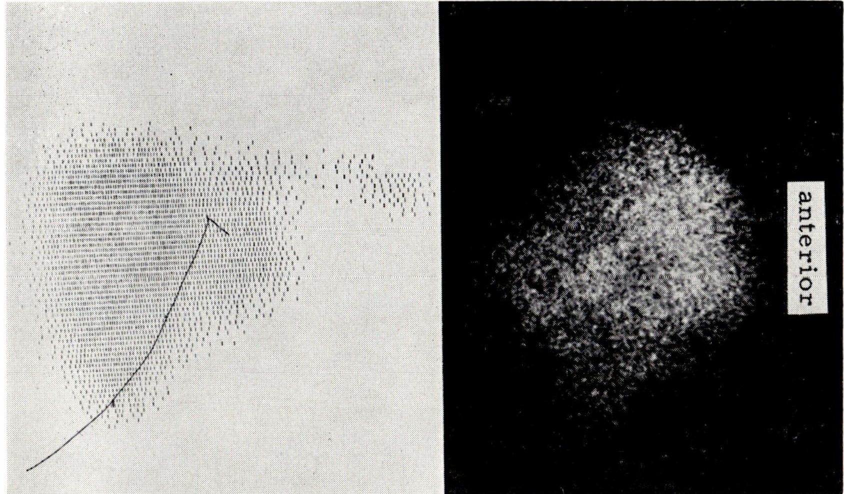

FIGURE 4-4. Frontal (*left*) and lateral (*right*) radiogold liver scans of a patient with breast carcinomatosis. The frontal projection of the liver appeared normal, but the degree of radiogold concentration in the spleen was higher than normally found with the level of background cut-off used on the rectilinear scanner. The lateral projection showed tumor destruction involving the posterior two-thirds of the right lobe. Lienal uptake was probably secondary to partial hepatic blood flow shunting through the tumor vascular bed, which is not lined with Kupffer cells. (Reproduced, courtesy of the *Journal of the Canadian Association of Radiologists, 17*:151, 1966.)

One of the pitfalls of radionuclide imaging devices is that a series of adjacent segments of tissue are monitored, and if the count rate of each segment is equal a uniform scan will be registered. Figure 4-5 is a frontal and lateral scan of a patient

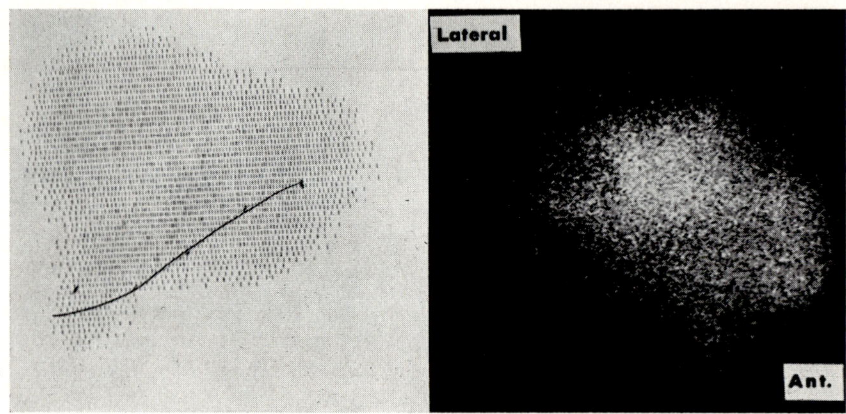

FIGURE 4-5. Frontal (*left*) and right lateral (*right*) radiogold liver scans in a patient with extensive focal replacement of liver substance by a colonic carcinoma. The frontal view appears normal, save for an indentation on the lateral margin, which may be a normal variation, but the right lateral scan portrays the true situation. Failure to see the lesions was not due to increased distance from the scintillation crystal, but rather to a fortuitously uniform count rate across the anterior liver surface. (Reproduced courtesy of the *Journal of the Canadian Association of Radiologists, 17*:151, 1966.)

with carcinoma of the sigmoid colon, and observed at laparotomy to have innumerable nodular deposits in the hepar. The frontal radiogold scan showed only an indentation of the right lateral margin, which could be a normal variation, but the lateral view demonstrated diffuse replacement from front to back.

Diffuse neoplastic involvement of the liver, as with malignant lymphomas, can be very difficult to detect. Hepatomegaly may be the only manifestation. A nebulous mottling of the radioactivity throughout the liver should be suspect in a patient with lymphoma. A return to uniformity, and/or reduction in size, following radiation therapy or chemotherapy is confirmatory (21).

NON-NEOPLASTIC DISEASES

Amoebic abscesses (19, 22, 23, 24) and hydatid cysts (25) present as hypoactive defects indistinguishable from neoplastic disease. However, Tandon *et al.* (23) were the only ones to report that the defects in amoebic abscesses appear to be covered with streaks of normal activity rendering a net-like pattern. They ascribe this to the fact that amoebic abscesses are traversed by trabecularly functioning cells which pick up the radioactive rose bengal, and are recorded as sparse strokes over the area of the functional defect. Multiple scans at different planes showed the presence of two or more amoebic abscesses in 27% of the cases.

If the biliary tree is sufficiently dilated, it may be reflected as a hypoactive area extending from the porta hepatis into the liver (26). Figure 4-6 is a frontal and lateral radiogold scan of a patient with a greatly dilated common duct and inflamed gall bladder, both of which were stuffed with radiolucent stones. The appearance is non-specific, but may be distinguished with

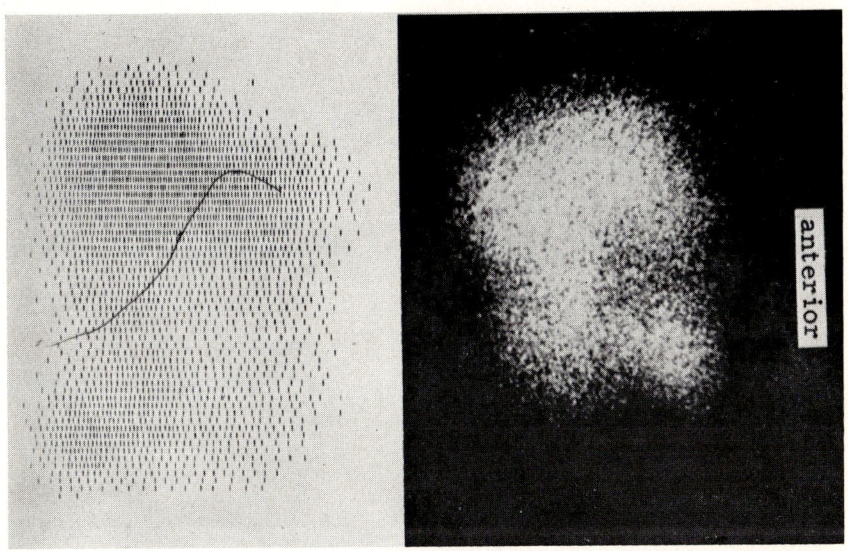

FIGURE 4-6. Frontal and lateral radiogold scans of a patient with stones in the gall bladder and common duct. The defect is caused by a greatly dilated choledochus.

serial radioactive rose bengal scans and observing a hyper-concentration within the distended biliary tree (27, 28, Chapter 5).

Polycystic liver disease presents with a number of well-delineated hypoactive defects, and simulates metastatic malignancy. However, the patient is usually in good health and the laboratory tests are normal (29).

Acute hepatitis may yield the so-called "salt and pepper" or "marblized" pattern with the radioactive rose bengal scan. This is due to poor uptake and subsequent low count rate, as the colloidal radiogold scan is uniform. Infrequently, the spleen may be seen to contain more than the normal complement of radiogold. In acute yellow atrophy, the liver may be seen to shrink in size. This is an ominous sign. Figure 4-7 represents radiogold hepatic scans obtained in a patient approximately one month apart. He was 57 years of age and jaundice developed shortly after surgery where Halothane was used as the anasthetic. The liver decreased in size between November 3rd and December 1st, and at the same time the 4.5-minute radiogold retention increased from a normal of 52% to 77%. Death interceded shortly afterward.

Christie and associates (30) claim that most of the diffuse

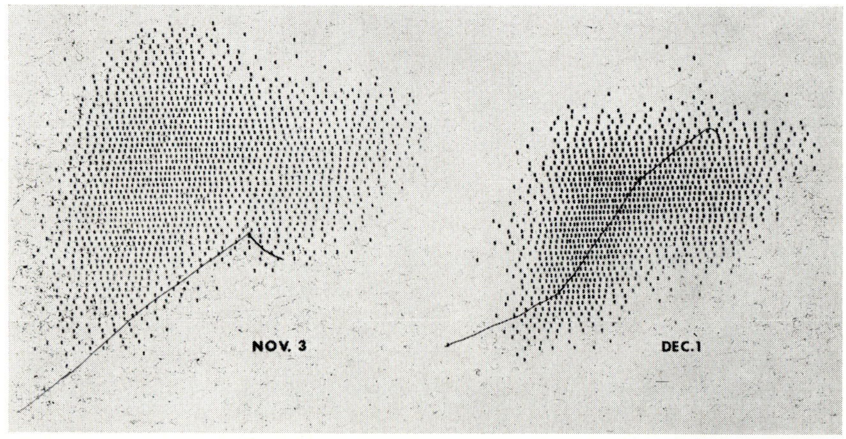

FIGURE 4-7.   Frontal radiogold scans on a patient with acute yellow atrophy taken November 3rd and December 1st. During this interval, the liver shrank in size, and the 4.5-minute radiogold retention increased from a normal of 52% to 77%.

irregularities seen in radiogold liver scans of patients with cirrhosis are due to insufficient count rate and statistical fluctuation. They found with serial background cut-off levels that the most active part of the liver is central and in the area of the hilar notch, and is not, as normally found, over the thicker right lobe. With progressive disease, there is a higher accumulation about the hilar notch plus visualization of the spleen. This is exemplified in Figure 4-8. The observed phenomenon is probably due to a diminished blood flow in the periphery of the liver, and apparently related to the increase in both portal and hepatic artery pressures, and to arterio-venous shunting which is known to be present in cirrhotic livers (30).

A large cirrhotic liver with focal areas of necrosis and regeneration, increased lienal uptake of radiogold, and elevated [131]I- rose bengal and radiogold retentions, can simulate extensive neoplastic replacement of the organ. Such a situation is exemplified in Figure 4-9 which represents the frontal and lateral radiogold scans obtained in a patient proved to have cirrhosis by liver biopsy and umbilical venography.

Castell and Johnson (31) evaluated portal systemic collateral

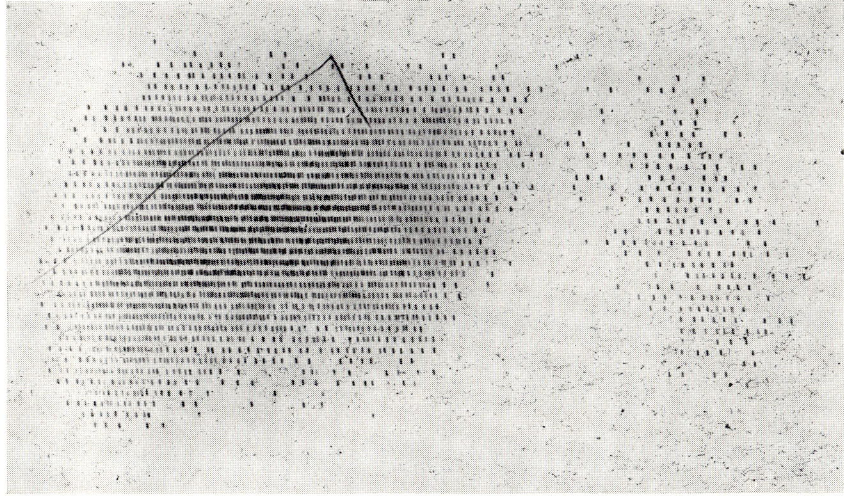

FIGURE 4-8. Colloidal [198]Au scan of a patient with nutritional cirrhosis. There is a higher concentration of radioactivity centrally, and a peripheral zone of relatively reduced concentration. The spleen has a higher than normal uptake of colloidal radiogold.

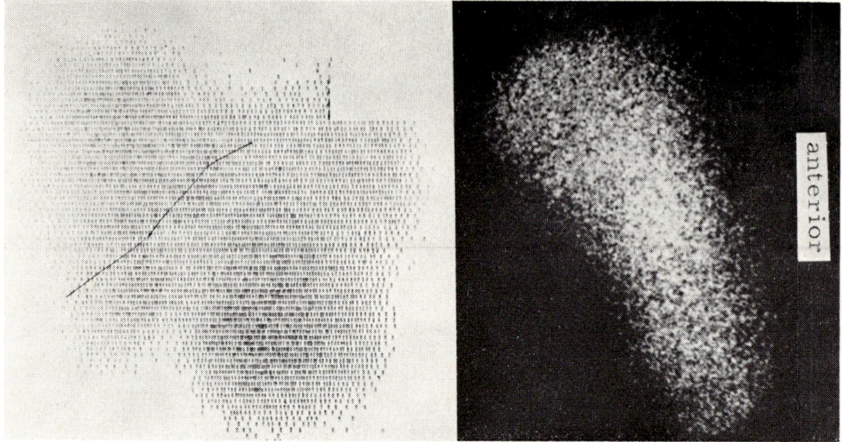

FIGURE 4-9.   Frontal (*left*) and lateral (*right*) colloidal radiogold liver scans of a patient with post-necrotic cirrhosis. The liver is enlarged and the multiple areas of reduced radiogold uptake render the appearance indistinguishable from diffuse involvement with neoplasia.

circulation in chronic liver disease by observing the degree of mottling of the radiogold deposition in the liver, and splenic and bone marrow uptake. The assessment was scored from 0 to $+3$ for each criterion, or a total value of 0 to $+9$. This was compared with the maximum arterial ammonia concentration obtained in an oral ammonia tolerance test. A linear relationship evolved with a correlation coefficient of 0.86. The correlation of each criterion separately was slightly less than the summation of the three. There is a direct correlation of the maximum arterial ammonia level with the degree of portal hypertension in cirrhotic patients.

The liver scan offers a good method of distinguishing a subphrenic abscess from intrathoracic disease. A combination lung-liver scan (32) will show a separation between the two organs in both a subphrenic abscess and loculated pleural fluid. However, peculiar to the subdiaphragmatic collection is a flattening and even depression of the dome surface of the liver. Figure 4-10 is a frontal and lateral view of a lung-liver scan obtained with radioiodinated macroaggregates of albumin and radiogold, respectively. The frontal projection portrays a wide separation between

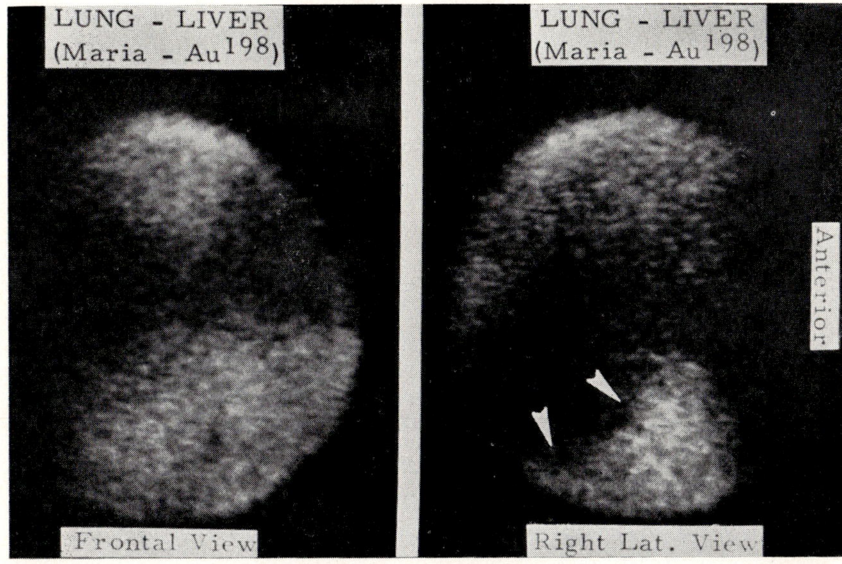

FIGURE 4-10.   A combined lung-liver scan obtained with the gamma-ray scintillation camera in a patient with a subdiaphragmatic abscess. The frontal view demonstrates a separation between the two organs, and the right lateral view shows, in addition, a depression of the dome surface of the liver (*arrows*).

the two organs, but on the right lateral scan the superior surface of the liver exhibits a concave outline. Approximately 800 ml of pus was subsequently drained.

Another example of a subdiaphragmatic abscess is illustrated in Figure 4-11. This 38-year-old male had a cholecystectomy, and developed signs and symptoms of an abscess postoperatively. He was refractory to antibiotic therapy. Subsequently the abdomen was entered via an anterior incision because the precise location of the abscess was unknown. A purulent collection could not be demonstrated at surgery. Three weeks later, a liver scan was requested for the first time. It clearly depicted an area of parenchymal replacement on the subdiaphragmatic surface of the right lobe on the frontal scan, but the lateral projection further localized it to the supero-dorsal area, beyond the peritoneal reflection. The abscess was then successfully drained through a posterior incision.

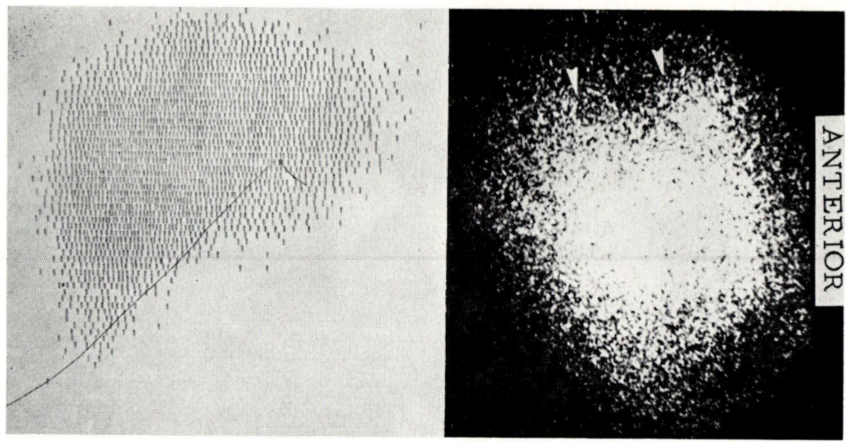

FIGURE 4-11.   A subphrenic abscess well localized on the lateral radiogold liver scan to the superoposterior surface (*arrow*). Prior anterior surgical exploration failed to locate it. The radionuclide study indicated the need for a posterior incision for drainage.

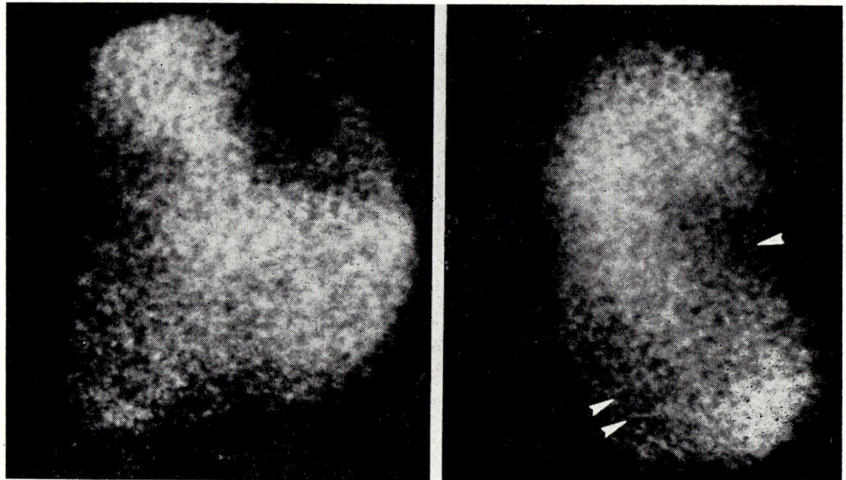

FIGURE 4-12.   Lung-liver scan obtained with ^{131}I macroaggregates of albumin and colloidal radiogold. The patient developed a subphrenic abscess following appendectomy. There is a reduced concentration in the right lobe of the liver, and a separation of the lung and liver laterally when viewed from the anterior projection (*left*). The lateral view (*right*) demonstrated a void anteriorly (*single arrow*), and posteriorly (*double arrows*). Two separated incisions were required for complete drainage.

A subphrenic abscess developed following an appendectomy in an 18-year-old female. The lung-liver scan (Fig. 4-12) showed a separation between the lateral half of the lung and liver on the frontal scan, plus a greatly diminished concentration of activity in the right hepatic lobe of the liver. On the lateral lung-liver scan a void was demonstrated anteriorly (*single arrow*) and posteriorly (*double arrows*). A posterior incision produced a large quantity of pus, but ameliorated the signs and symptoms minimally. Several days later, an anterior incision was productive of approximately 1,000 ml of fluid and the temperature promptly returned to normal. Apparently, there were two abscess pockets, and the radionuclide study functioned admirably in localizing them.

RADIATION INJURY

The histological effects of therapeutic doses of radiation have been described by Ogata *et al.* (33). These included arterial hyalinization, sinusoidal engorgement, desmoplasia, and atrophy and loss of polygonal cells. Ingold *et al.* (34) described a syndrome referred to as "Radiation Hepatitis" which consisted of hepatomegaly, ascites and jaundice. Thirteen out of 40 patients in whom the entire liver was irradiated to a dose exceeding 3,000 rads developed this condition, and three succumbed. Limited portions of the liver can be irradiated to doses as high as 5,500 rads without deleterious effects (35). Kurohara and co-workers (36) observed a segmental suppression of radioactive rose bengal and colloidal radiogold concentration in the liver corresponding to areas receiving a minimum of 3,000 rads in 30 days. The changes were at least partially reversible even after therapeutic doses of 4,520 rads provided the entire organ is not exposed to such a high level. The reticuloendothelial moiety appeared to be more radiosensitive than the polygonal cell component. Similar results were reported by Johnson *et al.* (37), who observed complete suppression of reticuloendothelial and parenchymal function within the irradiated sector of the liver seven to nine weeks after a dose as low as 2,400 rads in 20 days.

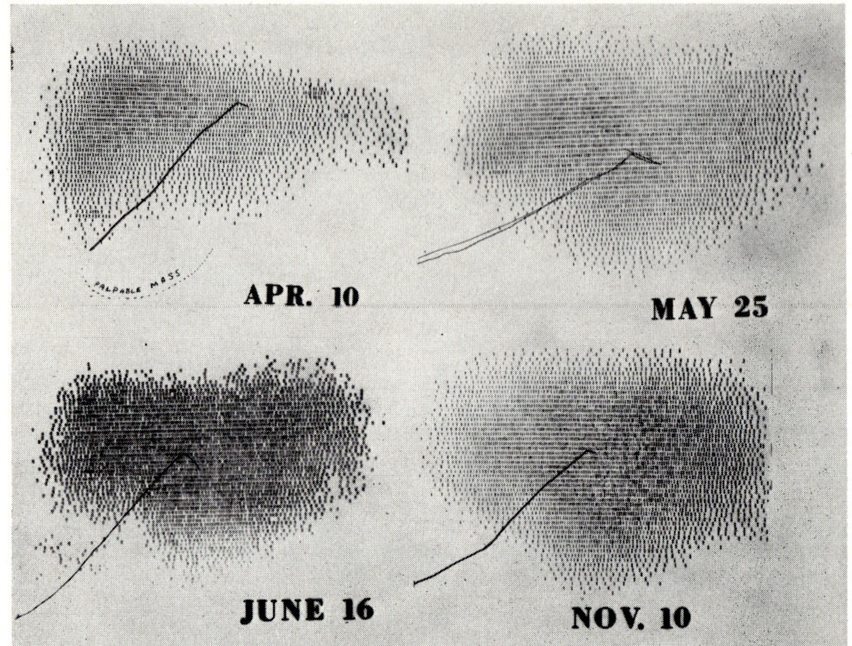

FIGURE 4-13. Serial radiogold liver scans in a patient with an hemangio-endothelial sarcoma. The scan obtained on April 10th had a normal configuration, but the palpable "mass" did not concentrate the radiogold, and therefore the scan was interpreted as being abnormal. On May 12th, a partial hepatectomy was performed. The scan on May 25th shows compensatory enlargement of the left lobe, which continued to grow until the last scan on November 10th. The latter demonstrates a greater concentration to the left of the xyphoid than to the right.

LIVER CONFIGURATION, POSITION AND SIZE

The shape of the liver is protean (14), both in its frontal and lateral projections, and requires considerable experience to avoid pitfalls in interpretation. Thus, a small or underdeveloped left lobe may be mistaken for tumor replacement, or a "beaver tail" type Riedel's lobe may be read as disease transecting the right lobe. Some consternation may accrue from a wide cleft in association with the falciform ligament, and the costal impression on the lateral aspect of the right lobe. Impression of a large hepatic vein on the superior surface, and the kidney indentation on the posterior surface of the right lobe might also be misinterpreted. It is imperative to examine the patient and transcribe onto the liver scan the lower edge of the liver or "mass," the right costal margin and xyphoid. If the palpated mass does not concentrate the test agent, then it is abnormal. A case in point is Figure 4-13 which represents serial colloidal radiogold scans of a patient with an hemangioendothelial sarcoma in the lower right lobe treated by partial hepatectomy. The preoperative scan showed a "normal" liver configuration, but a mass palpated in mid-respiration below the costal cage did not concentrate radiogold, and the scan was therefore interpreted as abnormal. Rapid compensatory regeneration of liver tissue, predominantly of the left lobe, is depicted in the post-hepatectomy scans.

A palpable liver is not necessarily an enlarged liver (38). It may be felt from 700 grams as weighed at necropsy, and yet be non-palpable and weigh as much as 2,800 grams (39). The liver volume relative to total body surface area is more meaningful than the absolute liver volume, and even this measurement has a poor correlation with clinical palpability (40).

The liver scan is admirably suited for determining both position and size, even in the presence of a rather rigid abdominal wall which resists examination, and in obese individuals. Figure 4-14 contains some representative examples. The upper left scan is a liver of normal size and shape, but whose edge was palpated "five finger-breadths" below the costal margin. A liver of similar size, configuration and position is shown in the upper right, but contains a tumor in the superior half of the right lobe. The liver exhibited in the lower left scan was felt "four finger-breadths" below the costal cage, and it was in fact enlarged, and harboured metastatic carcinoma in the right and left lobes. A patient with ovarian carcinoma was thought to have an abdomen full of metastatic deposits, but the scan, lower right, proved that it was an abdomen full of liver which in turn contained the bulk of the tumor.

In 1926, Pfahler attempted to establish a numerical basis for assessing hepatomegaly on the roentgenogram (41). He employed two measurements as indices of liver size. One of these was the distance from the highest point on the dome surface of the liver to the inferior tip of the right lobe, and the other from a point on the inferior surface of the right lobe, about midway between the vertical line through the xyphoid and the tip of the right lobe, to the region of the costophrenic angle (Fig. 4-15, lines A and B, respectively). The region of the costophrenic

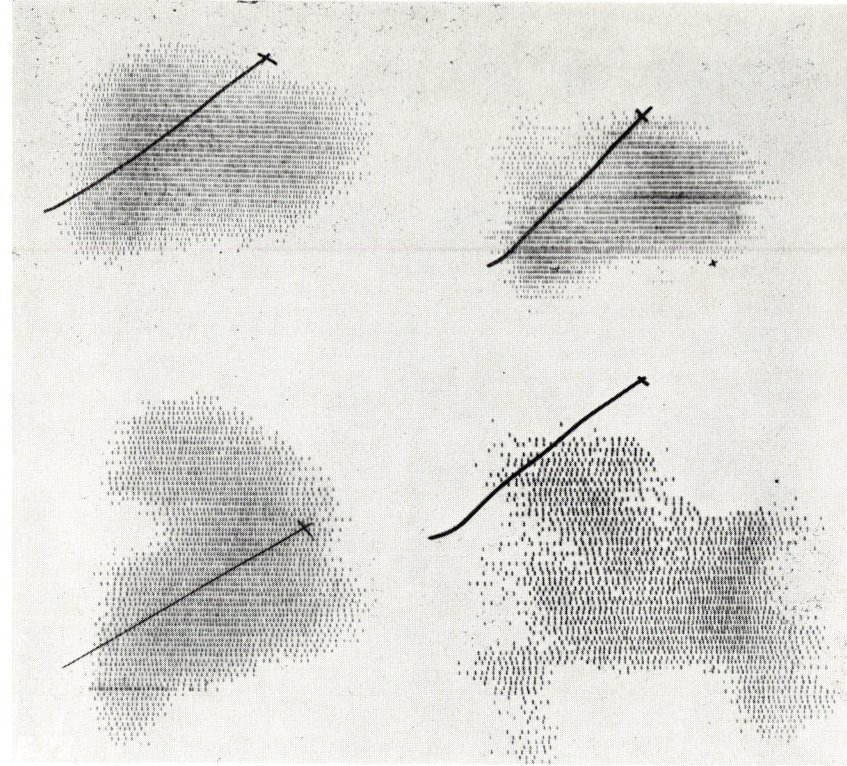

FIGURE 4-14. The distance between the palpable edge of the liver and costal margin is not necessarily an index of liver size. *Upper left*—Normal sized liver, but low lying. *Upper right*—Normal sized low-lying liver, but with tumor replacement of the superior half of the right lobe. The tumor was not palpable. *Lower left*—The liver lies below the costal margin to the same extent as those depicted in the upper left and upper right, but was also enlarged. Tumor replacement is observed in the right and left lobes. *Lower right*—This patient was thought to have an abdomen full of large deposits of ovarian carcinoma. The liver was not palpable. Findings on the scan revealed a greatly enlarged liver containing the bulk of the palpable tumor.

angle may be assumed to be the apex of the right lobe of the liver when the organ is lying on its inferior margin on a tabletop. At the 25-inch focal spot to film distance that Pfahler used, these values ranged from 18 to 22 cm for the distance A, and 14 to 19 cm for the distance B in normal adults. Transcribed to the

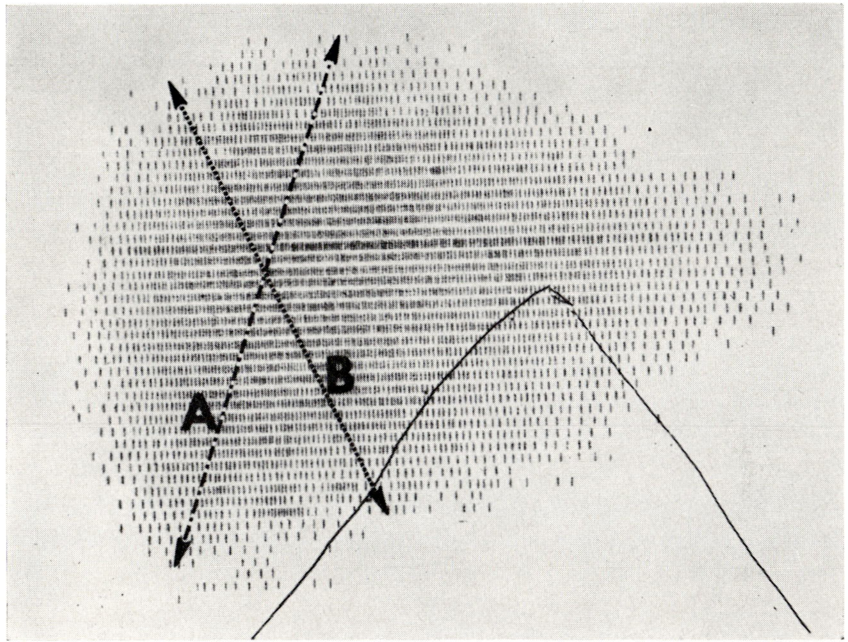

FIGURE 4-15. Pfahler's method of measuring liver size. Line A is drawn from the dome surface of the liver to the inferior tip of the right lobe. Line B is drawn from the inferior surface of the liver about midway between the vertical line through the xyphoid and the inferior tip of the right lobe, to the region of the costophrenic angle. The latter may be considered as the apex of the right lobe when the inferior surface is resting on a horizontal plane. The liver is considered enlarged when the sum of the measurements of A and B on the scan exceed 27 to 28 cm.

present-day usage of a 40-inch focal spot-film distance, the values are 16 to 20 cm and 12.5 to 17 cm, respectively. Keegan and Chase (42) found that Pfahler's parameters correlated better with the liver weight at autopsy than the projected area. They found that all livers which weighed more than 2,000 grams, and the majority weighing between 1,600 and 2,000 grams, had a sum of the two liver measurements exceeding 33 cm at a 40-inch focal spot-film distance. There were a few cases in which the sum was less than 33 cm, but the livers weighed more than the assumed normal of 1,400 grams. Extrapolating these results to the hepatic scan, where there is no appreciable magnification, combined measurements exceeding 27 to 28 cm reflect hepato-megaly. It is essentially a right lobe measurement, as the size of the left lobe does not enter into the calculation.

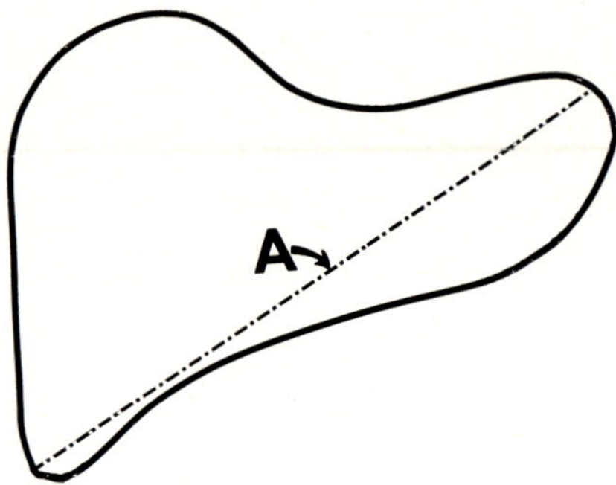

FIGURE 4-16. Walk's method of measuring liver size.
FIGURE 4-16A. *Frontal view.* Line A is the distance in centimeters be-tween the inferior tip of the right lobe and the most distal point on the left lateral border.

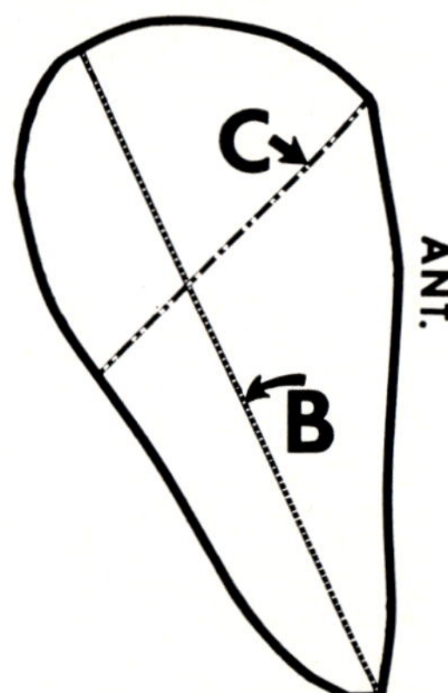

FIGURE 4-16B. *Right lateral view,* obliqued 30 degrees posteriorly. Line B is the distance in centimeters from the inferior tip of the right lobe to the most distal point on the postero-superior surface. Line C is the distance in centimeters from the posterior surface of the liver, where it lies adjacent to the upper pole of the kidney (about midway is a good approximation) to the junction of the anterior and dome surfaces of the liver.

$$\text{Liver volume in ml.} = \frac{A \times B \times C}{Index}$$

Walk (40) compared the liver volume, which was determined by measuring the amount of water displaced by the organ, with three linear measurements in 51 autopsied cases. He obtained the following relationship (Fig. 4-16):

$$\frac{A \times B \times C}{\text{Index}} = \text{Liver volume in ml.,}$$

where,   A is the true distance in cm between the inferior tip of the right lobe to the lateral border of the left lobe in the frontal projection.
       B is the true distance in cm between the inferior tip of the right lobe to the most distal length on the posterior surface in the lateral projection.
       C is the true distance in cm from the posterior surface of the liver where it lies close to the upper pole of the kidney (about midpoint), to the anterior costophrenic angle on the lateral projection.

The "index" varies somewhat with the configuration of the liver:

Liver Configuration	*Index* Range	*Mean*
Normal	3.0 to 4.1	3.55
Thin, flat right border	3.3 to 4.2	3.75
Blunt, thick right border	2.8 to 3.7	3.25

Walk emphasized that the liver lies obliquely in the abdomen, and in order to obtain true lateral dimensions the central ray of the x-ray beam must be angled 30 degrees posteriorly from the coronal plane, and, of course, it holds true for the liver scan as well. This point is well taken in Figure 4-17, A and B. Both are radiogold scans obtained with the gamma-ray scintillation camera. Figure 4-17A was taken with the patient lying supine and the detector head perpendicular to the sagittal plane on the right, and in Figure 4-17B the patient remained in the same position, but the detector head was angled 30 degrees posteriorly. Note the significant change in the C dimension, whereas B is not appreciably affected. The configuration observed in Figure 4-17A is due to the somewhat anterior lie of the left lobe relative to the right lobe. Walk claims an accuracy of 16% in his group of cases.

Normal relative liver volumes, that is, volume by mensuration divided by the body surface area (obtained from the DuBois tables, *Arch. Int. Med.*, 17:863, 1916) ranged from 550 to 860 ml. The liver was considered enlarged when the value exceeded 900 ml, and borderline between 800 and 900 ml.

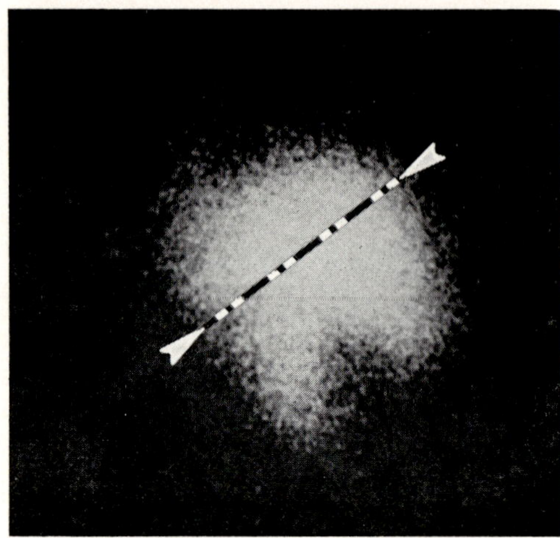

FIGURE 4-17A. Lateral colloidal radiogold liver scan in a supine patient with the detector normal to the sagittal plane.

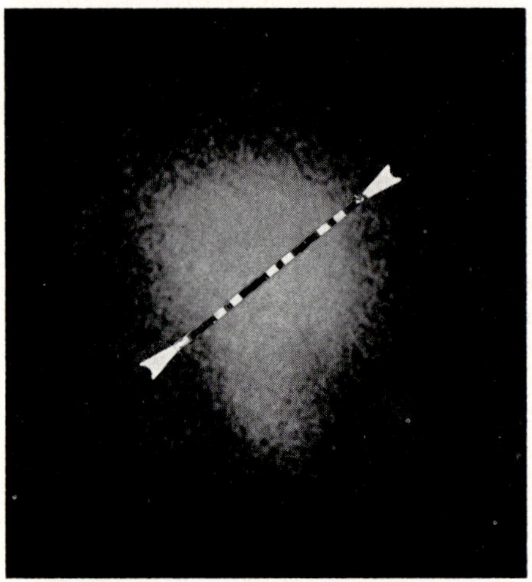

FIGURE 4-17B. To obtain the true right lateral projection of the liver the detector is angled 30° posteriorly.

ACCURACY OF LIVER SCANNING IN THE DETECTION OF DISEASE

Nagler and co-workers (44) were able to confirm the liver status in 548 scans. A correct interpretation was achieved in 461 patients, i.e., 84%. Of those patients who had tumor in the liver, 83% were correctly diagnosed, and 88% of the normal livers were read as such. The 69 patients with false-positive scans included such entities as cirrhosis, fatty metamorphosis, liver abscess, and liver necrosis with fatty metamorphosis. They found that the bromsulfalein retention and alkaline phosphatase to be the most consistently abnormal tests in patients with hepatic metastases.

A similar study was conducted by Gollin and associates (45). Some 380 liver scans performed on 357 patients were compared with the final diagnosis and results of liver function tests. The presence of focal disease on the scan was highly reliable, as there were only 2.5% false-positives. Alkaline phosphatase determinations were equally sensitive in detecting disease, but also rendered twice as many false-positives. The bromsulfalein test gave a higher number of abnormal results in established cases of focal disease, but the false positives were tenfold higher. Twenty-seven out of 101 cases with circumscribed hepatic lesions had their scans read as normal (27% false-negatives). The scan was weak in ferreting out diffuse disease, but, on the other hand, the liver function tests often failed to distinguish diffuse and localized disease, and they may be normal in the presence of large areas of focal parenchymal replacement. Over-all accuracy of the liver scan was 77%, and the alkaline phosphatase was next in order of reliability, followed by the bromsulfalein retention.

BIBLIOGRAPHY

1. Stirrett, L. A., Yuhl, E. T., and Libby, R. L.: A new technique for the diagnosis of carcinoma—metastatic—of the liver. *Surg., Gynec., & Obst.*, 96:210, 1953.

2. MacEwan, D. W.: Comparison of the uptake of radioactive iodinated human serum by liver tissue and liver metastases. *Am. J. Roentgenol., Rad. Therap. & Nucl. Med.*, 79:1001, 1958.

3. Stirrett, L. A., Yuhl, E. T., and Cassen, B.: Clinical applications of hepatic radioactivity surveys. *Am. J. Gastroenterology*, 21:310, 1954.

4. Ter-Pogossian, M., Kastner, J., and Vest, T. B.: Autofluorography of the thyroid gland by means of image amplification. *Radiology*, 81:984, 1963.

5. Anger, H. O.: Gamma ray and positron scintillation camera. *Nucleonics*, 21:52, 1963.

6. BENDER, M. A., AND BLAU, M.: Autofluoroscope. *Nucleonics,* 21:52, 1963.

7. TAPLIN, G. V., DORE, E. K., AND JOHNSON, D. E.: Clinical studies of reticuloendothelial function with colloidal suspensions of human albumin I[131]. *USAEC Report UCLA-289,* 1961.

8. HARPER, P. V., LATHROP, K. A., AND McCARDLE, R. J.: Improved liver scanning with 6-hour Tc[99]m in fat emulsion. *J. Nuclear Med.,* 4:189, 1963.

9. DWORKIN, H. J., NELIS, A., AND DOWSE, L.: Rectilinear liver scanning with technetium-99m sulfide colloid. *Am. J. Roentgenol., Rad. Therap. & Nucl. Med., 101*:557, 1967.

10. HARPER, P. V., LATHROP, K. A., AND RICHARDS, P.: Tc-99m as a radiocolloid. *J. Nuclear Med., 5*:382, 1964.

11. GOODWIN, D. A., STERN, H. S., AND WAGNER, H. N.: A new radiopharmaceutical for liver scanning. *Nucleonics, 24*:65, 1966.

12. JOHNSTON, G. S., HUPF, H. B., GOTSHALL, E., AND KYLE, R. A.: Zinc 69m chloride: A new liver scanning agent. *Am. J. Roentgenol., Rad. Therap. & Nucl. Med., 101*:548, 1967.

13. CHRISTIE, J. H., AND MacINTYRE, W. J.: Liver scanning. In, *Progress in Medical Radioisotope Scanning.* Edited by R. M. KNISELEY, *et al.* U. S. Atomic Energy Commission, T.I.D., 7673:405, 1962.

14. WAGNER, H. N., McAFEE, J. G., AND MOZLEY, J. M.: Diagnosis of liver disease by radioisotope scanning. *A.M.A. Arch. Int. Med., 107*:324, 1961.

15. OZARDA, A., AND PICKREN, J.: Topographic distribution of liver metastases: Its relation to surgical and isotope diagnosis. *J. Nuclear Med., 3*:149, 1962.

16. SCHUMAN, B. M., BLOCK, M. A., EYLER, W. R., AND DuSAULT, L.: Liver abscess: Rose bengal I[131] hepatic photoscan in diagnosis and management. *J.A.M.A., 187*:708, 1964.

17. BONTE, F. J., KROHMER, J. S., ELMENDORF, E., PRESLEY, N. L., AND ANDREWS, G. J.: Scintillation scanning of liver. II. Clinical applications. *Am. J. Roentgenol., Rad. Therap. & Nucl. Med., 88*:275, 1962.

18. LOKEN, M. K., AND GERDING, D.: Visualization of filling defects in a liver phantom containing Tc[99]m, Hg[197], I[131] or Au[198] using a rectilinear scanner or scintillation camera. *Am. J. Roentgenol., Rad. Therap. & Nucl. Med., 101*:551, 1967.

19. CZERNIAK, P., BANK, H., AND PAUZNER, Y.: Radioisotopic scanning in liver echinococcosis. *Radiology, 83*:690, 1964.

20. ROSENTHALL, L., AND USHER, M. S.: Assessment of combined frontal and lateral views in liver scanning. *Journal, Can. Assoc. Radiologists, 17*:151, 1966.

21. MOLANDER, D. W., ARIEL, I. M., AND PACK, G. T.: Hepatic gamma

scanning as an aid in the management of patients with malignant lymphomas. *Am. J. Roentgenol., Rad. Therap. & Nucl. Med.,* 99:851, 1967.

22. TURRILL, F. L., AND BURNHAM, J. R.: Hepatic amebiasis. *Am. J. Surg.,* 111:424, 1966.

23. TANDON, B. N., CHOUDHURY, A. K. R., TIKARE, S. K., AND WIG, K. L.: A study of hepatic amebiasis by radioactive rose bengal scanning of the liver. *Am. J. Tropical Med. & Hygiene,* 15:16, 1966.

24. CUARON, A., SEPULVEDA, B., AND LANDA, L.: Topographic distribution of amoebic abscesses studied by liver scanning. *Internat. J. Appl. Radiation and Isotopes,* 16:603, 1965.

25. MORRIS, J., DOUST, B., AND HANKS, T.: The roentgenologic and radioisotopic assessment of hydatid disease of the liver. *Am. J. Roentgenol., Rad. Therap. & Nucl. Med.,* 101:519, 1967.

26. MORRIS, J., MCRAE, J., PERKINS, K. W., AND ARTER, W.: Liver scanning in obstructive jaundice using colloidal radiogold. *J. Coll. Radiol. Australasia,* 9:68, 1965.

27. EYLER, W. R., SCHUMAN, B. M., DU SAULT, L. A., AND HINSON, R. E.: The radioiodinated rose bengal liver scan as an aid in the differential diagnosis of jaundice. *Am. J. Roentgenol., Rad. Therap. & Nucl. Med.,* 94:469, 1965.

28. ROSENTHALL, LEONARD: The application of colloidal radiogold and radioiodinated rose bengal in hepatobiliary disease. *Am. J. Roentgenol., Rad. Therap. & Nucl. Med.,* 101:561, 1967.

29. PELTOKALLIO, P., TASKINEN, P. J., AND PELTOKALLIO, V.: The value of liver scanning in the diagnosis of polycystic disease of the liver. *Am. J. Roentgenol., Rad. Therap. & Nucl. Med.,* 101:543, 1967.

30. CHRISTIE, J. H., MACINTYRE, W. J., CRESPO, G. G., AND KOCH-WESER, D. E.: Radioisotope scanning in hepatic cirrhosis. *Radiology,* 81:455, 1963.

31. CASTELL, D. O., AND JOHNSON, R. B.: The [198]Au liver scan. An index of portal-systemic collateral circulation in chronic liver disease. *new Eng. J. Med.,* 275:188, 1966.

32. BROWN, D. W.: Lung-liver scans in diagnosis of sub-diaphragmatic abscess. *J.A.M.A.,* 197:728, 1966.

33. OGATA, K., HIZAWA, K., YOSHIDA, M., KITAMURO, T., AGATI, G., KAGAWA, K., AND FUKADA, F.: Hepatic injury following irradiation— Morphologic study. *Tokushima J. Exp. Med.,* 9:240, 1963.

34. INGOLD, J. A., REED, G. D., KAPLAN, H. S., AND BAGSHAW, M. A.: Radiation hepatitis. *Am. J. Roentgenol., Rad. Therap. & Nucl. Med.,* 93:200, 1965.

35. CONCANNON, J. P., EDELMAN, A., FRICH, J. C., AND KUNKEL, G.: Localized "radiation hepatitis" as demonstrated by scintillation scanning. *Radiology,* 89:136, 1967.

36. KUROHARA, S. S., SWENSON, N. L., USSELMAN, J. A., AND GEORGE, F. W.: Response and recovery of liver to radiation as demonstrated by photoscans. *Radiology*, 89:129, 1967.

37. JOHNSON, P. M., GROSSMAN, F. M., AND ATKINS, H. L.: Radiation induced hepatic injury. *Am. J. Roentgenol., Rad. Therap. & Nucl. Med.*, 99:453, 1967.

38. PALMER, E. D.: Palpability of the liver edge in healthy adults. *U. S. Armed Forces M. J.*, 9:1685, 1958.

39. ZELMAN, S.: Liver and spleen visualization by a simple roentgen contrast method. *Ann. Int. Med.*, 34:466, 1951.

40. WALK, L.: Roentgenologic determination of the liver volume. *Acta Radiologica*, 55:49, 1961.

41. PFAHLER, G. E.: The measurement of the liver by means of roentgen rays: Based upon a study of 502 subjects. *Am. J. Roentgenol., Rad. Therap. & Nucl. Med.*, 16:558, 1926.

42. KEEGAN, A., AND CHASE, N.: In, *Roentgenology of the Abdomen*, by Juan Taveras and Ross Golden. The Williams and Wilkins Company, Baltimore, 1961, pp 14:109.

43. YAGAN, R., MACINTYRE, W. J., AND CHRISTIE, J. H.: Estimation of liver size by the multiple cut off scintillation scanning technique. *Am. J. Roentgenology, Rad. Therap. & Nucl. Med.*, 88:289, 1962.

44. NAGLER, W., BENDER, M. A., AND BLAU, M.: Radioisotope photoscanning of the liver. *Gastroenterology*, 44:36, 1963.

45. GOLLIN, F. F., SIMS, J. L., AND CAMERON, J. R.: Liver scanning and liver function tests. *J.A.M.A.*, 187:111, 1964.

Chapter 5

THE USE OF RADIOIODINATED ROSE BENGAL CLEARANCE, AND SERIAL LIVER AND ABDOMINAL SCANNING TO DIFFERENTIATE EXTRAHEPATIC OBSTRUCTIVE JAUNDICE AND INTRAHEPATIC DISEASE

SERIAL SCANS OF A normal liver and abdomen following an intravenous dose of about 200 microcuries ^{131}I- rose bengal will show a uniform distribution within the liver, and with time a uniform drainage from the organ into the gall bladder and gut. Maximum hepatic uptake occurs at 20 minutes, and the activity in the cardiac blood pool, which reflects the background, levels off to a minimum at approximately 30 minutes. Accumulation in the gall bladder and small bowel may be observed as early as 25 minutes (1). In the presence of intrahepatic disease and obstructive choledochopathy, these time relationships are altered. However, dependence upon the time of arrival of radioactive dye in the gut or the qualitative assessment of its concentration in the cardiac blood pool is not always a reliable means of distinguishing polygonal cell disease, and partial and complete extrahepatic biliary obstruction. A correlation of the radioactive rose bengal retention, its distribution within the liver, and the presence or absence of it in the bowel is more fruitful (2). An assessment restricted to the liver distribution and activity levels in the gut only has been reported by Eyler *et al.* (3, 4) and Shehadi (5).

TECHNIQUE

The patient is positioned supine and a scintillation detector with a twenty degree divergent collimator is placed against the side of the head, encompassing the ear. A rate meter and strip chart recorder are linked to the probe. An intravenous injection of 200 microcuries ^{131}I rose bengal is administered, and the head is monitored continuously for 20 minutes. A 20-minute retention is obtained from the ratio of the net 20-minute count rate to the 5-minute count rate off the tracing (see Chapter 2). The liver and abdomen are then scanned at 30 minutes, 3 hours, 6 hours and 24 hours. Finally, a colloidal radiogold scan is performed to compare the distribtuion of the two radiopharmaceuticals.

UNIFORM LIVER AND NO EXCRETION INTO THE GUT

The presence of a uniform distribution of radioactive dye in the liver and no detectable excretion into the gut is associated with three possible entities. If the 20-minute retention of ^{131}I-rose bengal is greater than 86%, it is virtually pathognomonic of polygonal cell disease, whether or not activity is observed in the bowel. In fact, only two cases of primary polygonal cell disease were encountered which had no detectable bile excretion, but were associated with 20 minute retentions of 100%. An example of a patient with acute hepatitis and a bilirubin of 14 mg per cent is shown in Figure 5-1. The 20-minute retention was 91%, and although the scan at 20 minutes showed an understandably low uptake in the liver, it was uniform and remained homogeneous at 3 and 24 hours. The gall bladder was first observed at 3 hours, and persisted at 24 hours, but more importantly, is the definite accumulation of radioactive dye in the right colon, which rules out a complete obstruction.

Complete obstruction is associated with an [131]I- rose bengal retention of 86%, or less, and no activity in the gut. It is essential to distinguish radioactivity in the kidneys and urinary vesical from the bowel. The presence of radioactive dye in the kidneys can be found in either hepatocellular or obstructive jaundice. A patient with carcinoma of the head of the pancreas and complete obstruction of the common duct is depicted in Figure 5-2. The 20-minute retention was 82%. There is no evidence of bile excre-

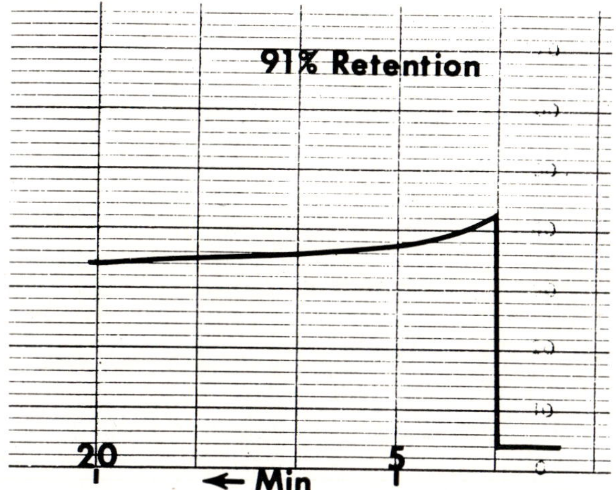

FIGURE 5-1. A patient with acute hepatitis, and a serum bilirubin of 14 mg %.

FIGURE 5-1A. Twenty-minute ^{131}I- rose bengal retention of 91%.

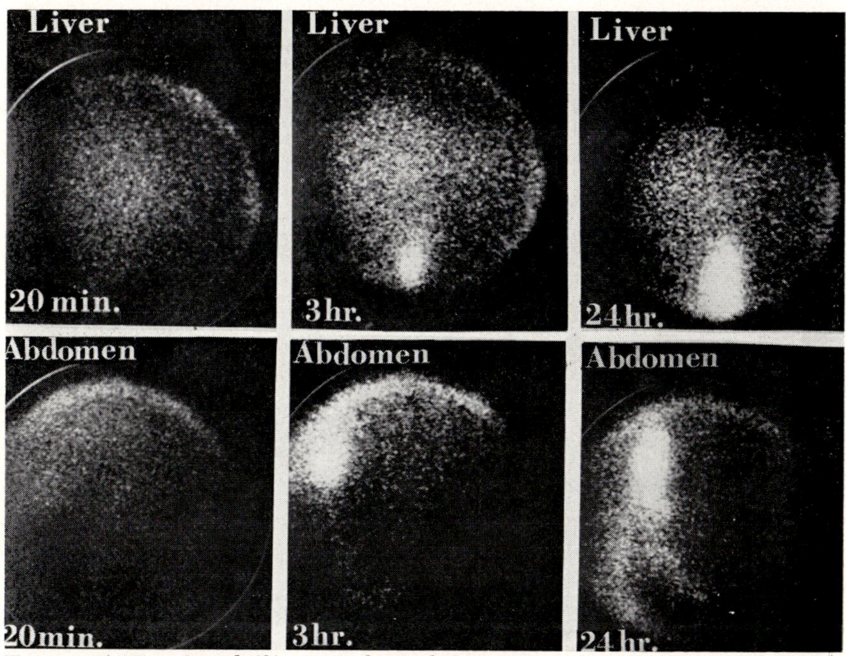

FIGURE 5-1B. Serial ^{131}I- rose bengal scans started immediately after the retention study. The distribution of radioactivity remains uniform within the liver; the gall bladder is visualized, and radioactive is present in the ascending and transverse colon at 24 hours.

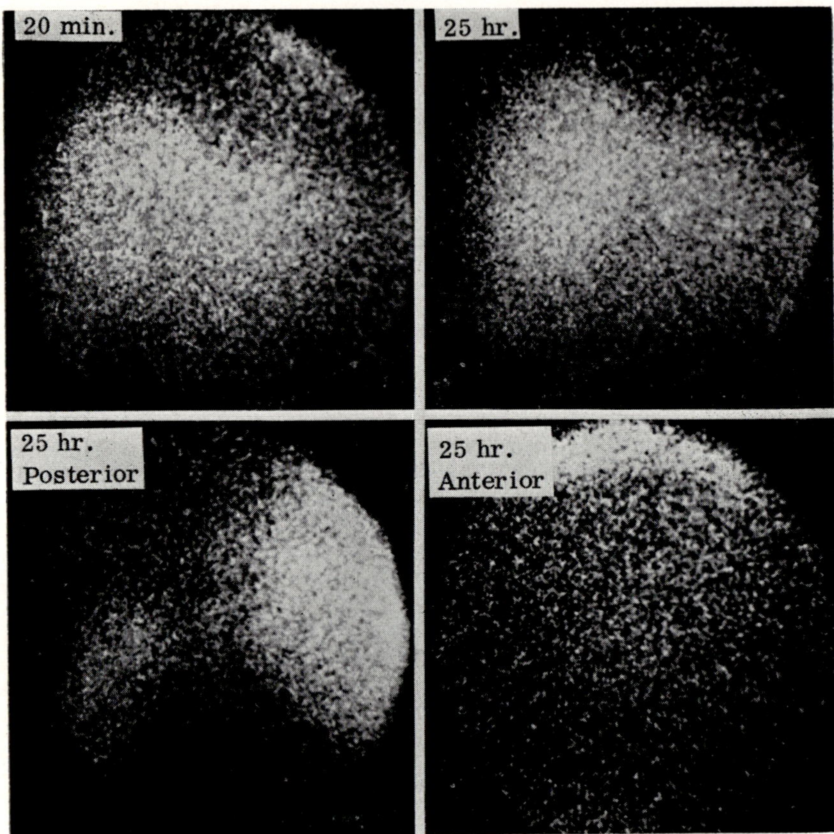

FIGURE 5-2.   A patient with complete choledocal obstruction secondary to carcinoma of the head of the pancreas. At 24 hours, no radioactive rose bengal is observed in the bowel. The kidneys are well demonstrated in the posterior scan, and should not be confused with biliary excretion of the test agent.

tion on the 25-hour anterior abdominal scan, but from the posterior projection the kidneys are well outlined.

In toxic hepatitis, due to Chlorpromazine, cancer chemotherapeutic drugs, etc., the distribution of activity in the liver is homogeneous, the ^{131}I- rose bengal retention is less than 86%, and there is excretion into the gut. One case out of 7 did not show activity in the bowel within a 24 hour interval. She was a mental patient on Chlorpromazine, and the 20-minute retention was 72%. Thus, when there is no bile excretion distinction from complete extrahepatic obstruction on the basis of the radio-nuclide study alone is impossible. In the presence of bile excretion into the bowel and a uniform distribution of activity in the liver, toxic hepatitis resembles hepatocellular disease and partial extrahepatic obstruction, unless the latter condition shows evidence of ^{131}I rose bengal accumulating in a dilated biliary tree.

If the ^{131}I- rose bengal retention is between 80 and 86%, distribution of activity in the liver is uniform, and excretion of radioactivity is present, then this usually denotes hepatocellular disease. Obstructive jaundice with retentions between 80 and 86% are generally complete, and uncomplicated partial obstructions have retentions less than 80%.

INCREASED CONCENTRATION IN THE REGION OF THE PORTA HEPATIS

An increase in the concentration of ^{131}I- rose bengal in the region of the porta hepatis, and extending into the liver, is due to the radioactive dye accumulating in a dilated biliary duct system. This is the hallmark of partial choledochal obstruction when radioactive dye is seen in the bowel within 24 hours. Otherwise, the differentiation of acute hepatitis, intrahepatic cholestatic jaundice and partial extrahepatic obstruction cannot be made. Figure 5-3 represents a radioactive rose bengal series in a 75-year-old female with carcinoma of the head of the pancreas. The 20-minute rose bengal retention was 65%, 4.5-minute radiogold retention 56%, bilirubin 3.3 mg per cent, alkaline phosphatase 82, serum glutamic oxaloacetic transaminase (SGOT) 22, and serum glutamic pyruvic transaminase (SGPT) 20. At 6 hours, there is an increased concentration of radioactive dye extending into the liver from the region of the porta hepatis, and it stands out in greater relief at 24 hours. Activity is seen in the small bowel at 6 hours, and in the large bowel at 24 hours, indicating partial choledochal obstruction. At autopsy the diameter of the common bile duct was 1.5 cm.

Another patient with partial obstruction due to carcinoma of the pancreas is illustrated in Figure 5-4. At 1 hour, the radioactive rose bengal scan demonstrated a hypoactive area adjacent to the porta hepatis. By 3 hours this region filled in, and was

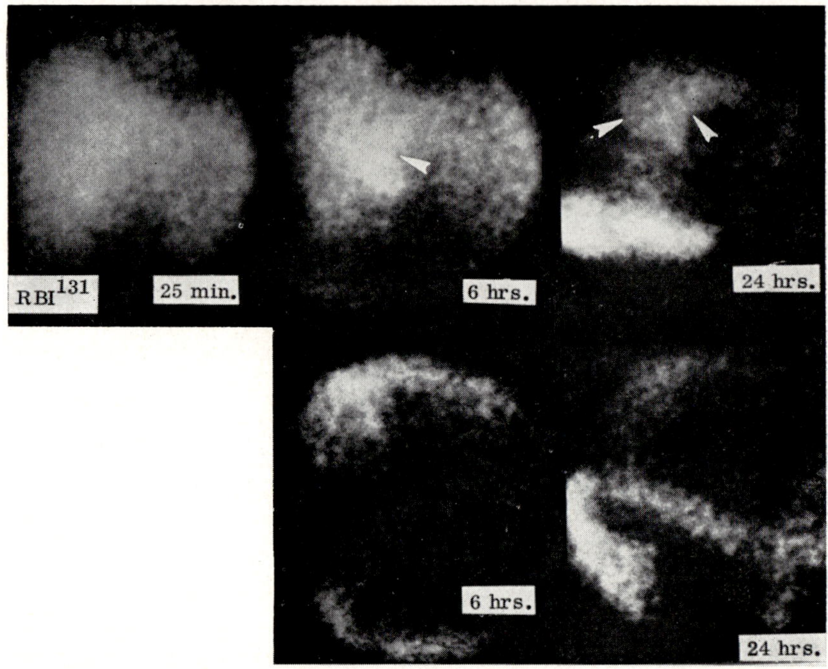

FIGURE 5-3. A 75-year-old female with carcinoma of the head of the pancreas partially obstructing the common duct. At 25 minutes, the distribution of ^{131}I- rose bengal in the liver is uniform, but at 6 and 24 hours there is an accumulation of radioactive material in the dilated biliary duct system (*arrows*). Excretion is observed at 6 hours, and by 24 hours the radioactivity is largely confined to the colon.

of the same concentration as the rest of the organ. This presumably was due to delayed excretion into the dilated biliary ducts. A modicum of radioactive dye is seen in the abdomen at 3 hours, substantiating the incompleteness of the obstruction, which was verified at laparotomy.

The following study was obtained in a patient confined to a mental institution and medicated with large doses of Chlorpromazine. She developed a painless, deep icterus, and had obstructive blood chemistries. The differential diagnosis rested between Chlorpromazine toxic hepatitis and extrahepatic obstructive jaundice. There was a good uptake of radioactive rose bengal as reflected by a 20-minute retention of 75%, and a low back-

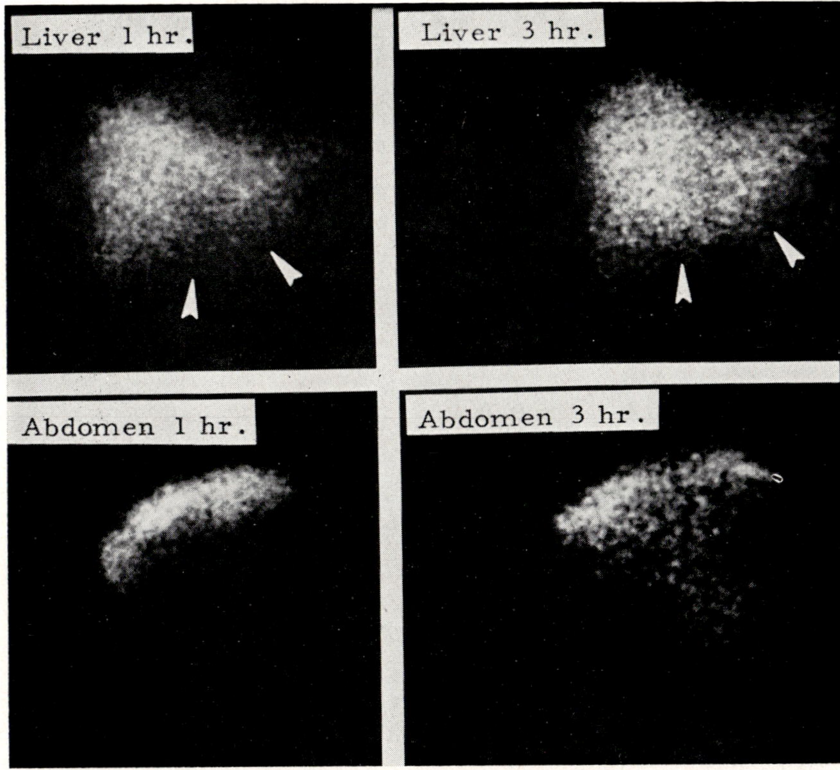

FIGURE 5-4. Partial choledochal obstruction due to carcinoma of the pancreas was established at laparotomy in this patient. The ^{131}I- rose bengal series showed a reduction in concentration in the region of the porta hepatis at 1 hour, but at 3 hours the area filled in (*arrows*). Early biliary excretion is observed at 3 hours in the scan of the abdomen.

ground at 30 minutes on the liver scan. However, the 30-minute liver scan exhibited a peripheral zone of reduced activity relative to the central two-thirds. By 6 hours, this central zone shifted toward the porta hepatis and decreased in size. At 24 hours, the situation was not significantly changed (Fig. 5-5A). The large bowel distal to the hepatic flexure contained radioactive dye at 24 hours, and thus established a diagnosis of partial extrahepatic common duct obstruction. A transhepatic cholangiogram (Fig. 5-5B) demonstrated a stone impacted in the distal end of the common duct and obstructing it completely. The biliary tree

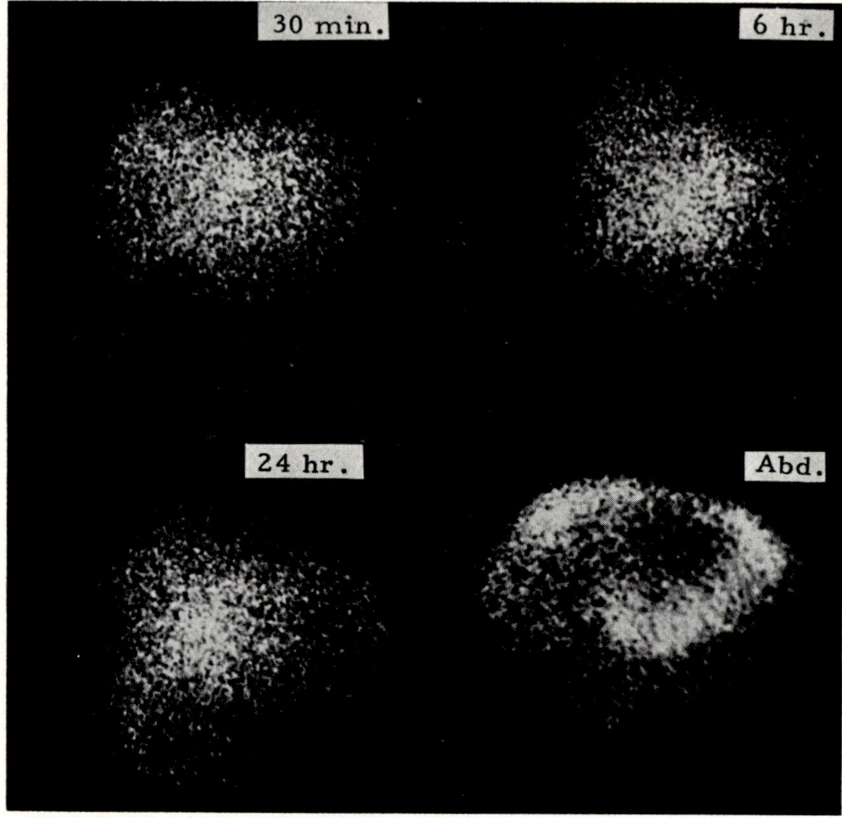

FIGURE 5-5.   Serial ^{131}I- rose bengal scans in a patient deeply jaundiced and on large doses of chlorpromazine.

FIGURE 5A.   At 30 minutes, there is a higher concentration of radioactive material in the central two-thirds of the liver, which contracts in size toward the porta hepatis at 6 and 24 hours. The abdominal scan at 24 hours depicts activity in the large bowel distal to the hepatic flexure, thus establishing a diagnosis of partial extrahepatic obstructive jaundice.

proximally was greatly dilated, but there was an unusual choledocho-colonic fistula, which accounted for the radioactive dye in the colon. In retrospect, this could be seen in the 24 hour abdominal scan, but it could not have been diagnosed prospectively unless short interval scans were obtained and colon activity observed to the exclusion of the small bowel.

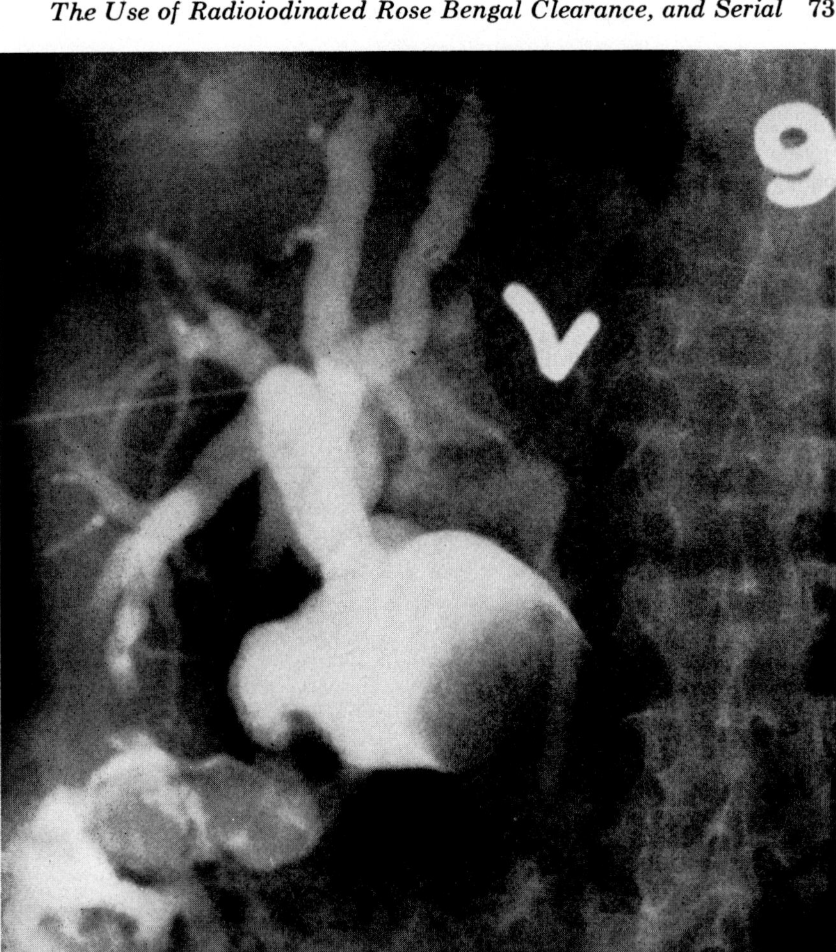

FIGURE 5B. Transhepatic cholangiogram showing a dilated biliary tree and a large stone impacted in the distal end of the common duct obstructing it completely. However, there is a choledocho-colonic fistula accounting for the [131]I- bengal in the transverse colon.

NON-UNIFORM DRAINAGE FROM THE LIVER

A non-uniform drainage of radioactive rose bengal from the liver can be caused by partially obstructing stones in the biliary radicals. The scans in Figures 5-6, A and B, were taken at 45

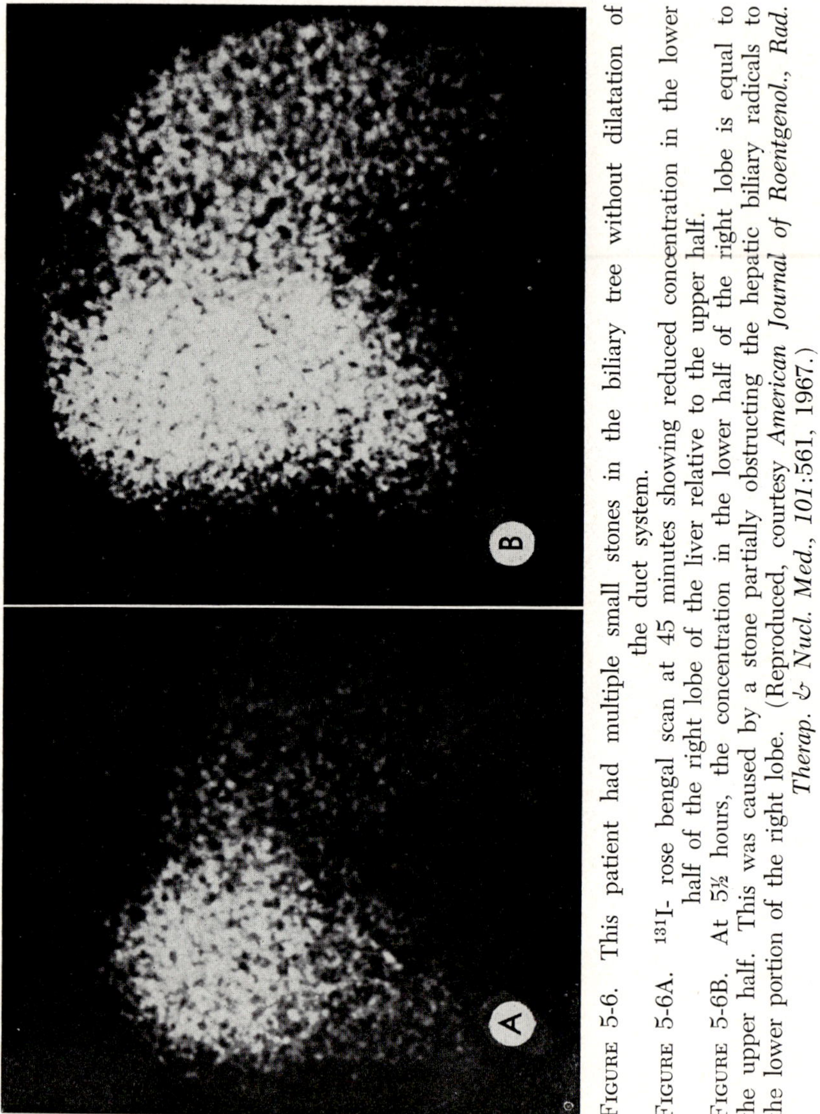

FIGURE 5-6. This patient had multiple small stones in the biliary tree without dilatation of the duct system.

FIGURE 5-6A. ^{131}I- rose bengal scan at 45 minutes showing reduced concentration in the lower half of the right lobe of the liver relative to the upper half.

FIGURE 5-6B. At 5½ hours, the concentration in the lower half of the right lobe is equal to the upper half. This was caused by a stone partially obstructing the hepatic biliary radicals to the lower portion of the right lobe. (Reproduced, courtesy *American Journal of Roentgenol., Rad. Therap. & Nucl. Med., 101:*561, 1967.)

minutes and 5½ hours respectively, in a 61-year-old female who was found to have multiple stones in the choledochus and both hepatic biliary ducts, but no distention. The bilirubin was 1.4 mg per cent and the 20-minute rose bengal retention 63%. At 45 minutes, there was less activity in the lower half of the right lobe than in the upper half. At 5½ hours, the concentration in the two halves was equal. This change was presumably caused by a stone partially obstructing the hepatic biliary radicals to the lower portion of the right lobe.

PERSISTENT HYPOACTIVE AREAS WITH ^{131}I- ROSE BENGAL AND COLLOIDAL RADIOGOLD

Persistent areas of reduced or absent activity in the liver with the ^{131}I- rose bengal series and radiogold usually denote space occupying disease as opposed to a dilated biliary tree. This is true whether or not there is excretion into the gut, and no matter what the 20-minute ^{131}I- rose bengal retention reads. The odd case of partial extrahepatic obstructive jaundice presents itself with a uniform distribution of radioactive rose bengal, but the colloidal radiogold scan portrays a hypoactive area corresponding to a dilated biliary duct system.

INDETERMINATE GROUP

This category includes those patients with radioactive rose bengal retentions less than 80%, a uniform distribution of activity within the liver and excretion into the intestines. Partial extrahepatic obstruction, mild-to-moderate hepatitis and intrahepatic cholestatic jaundice can all yield this picture.

A summary of the results of ^{131}I- rose bengal (^{131}IRB) and serial liver scans is given in the following table:

^{131}IRB Retention (%)	Excretion into Gut in 24 hrs.	Distribution of ^{131}IRB in the Liver	Diagnosis
86-100	+ ve or − ve	Uniform	Polygonal cell disease
> 80	+ ve	Uniform	Polygonal cell disease
⩽ 86	− ve	Uniform or increased in region of porta hepatis.	Complete extrahepatic biliary obstruction.
⩽ 80	+ ve	Increased in region of porta hepatis or non-uniform drainage.	Partial biliary obstruction
> 45	+ ve or − ve	Persistent hypoactive areas with ^{131}IRB and ^{198}Au.	Intrahepatic lesion.
< 80	+ ve	Uniform	Indeterminate

DETECTION OF BILE PERITONITIS

Serial radioactive rose bengal scans may sometimes be helpful

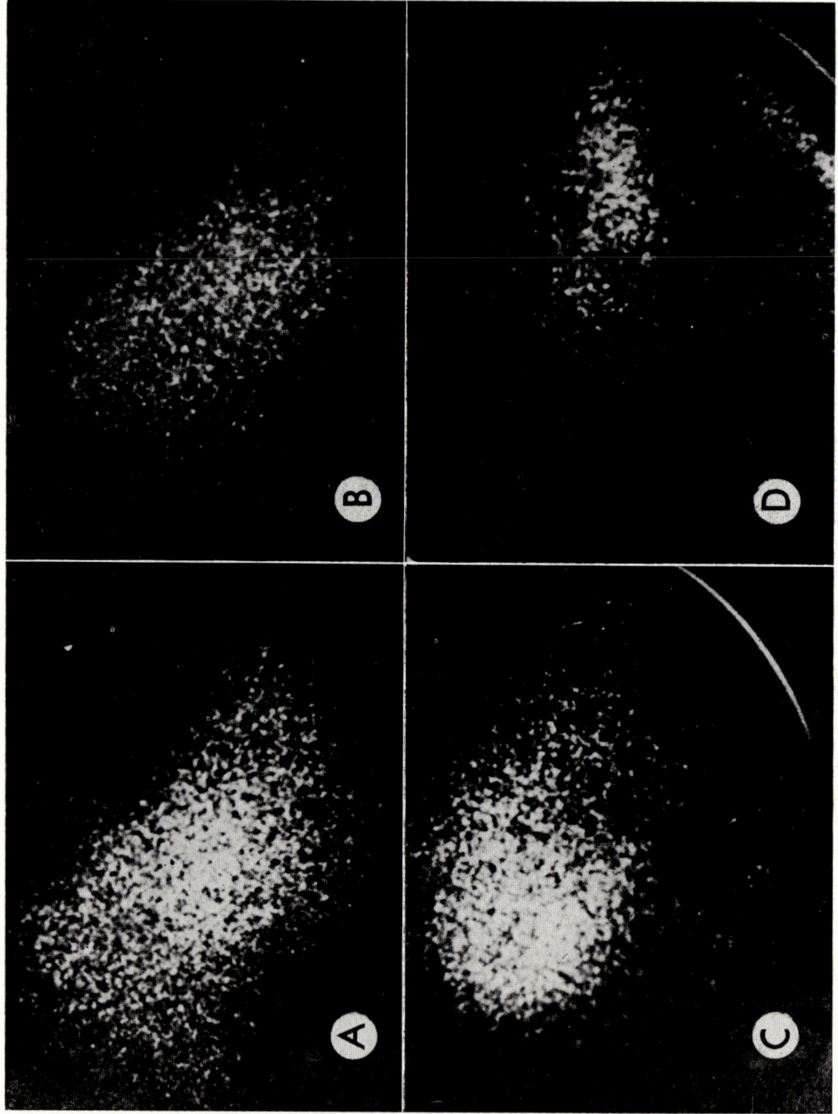

FIGURE 5-7.　An 80-year-old male with carcinoma of the biliary ducts and extension into the right lobe of the liver. Serial [131]I- rose bengal liver scans at 4 and 24 hours show a progressively increasing concentration of activity over the right lobe of the liver. This was due to a bile leak extending over the surface of the liver. Radioactive material is demonstrated in the transverse colon as well at 24 hours. (Reproduced, courtesy of the *Am. J. Roentgenol. Rad. Therap. & Nucl. Med., 101*:561, 1967.)

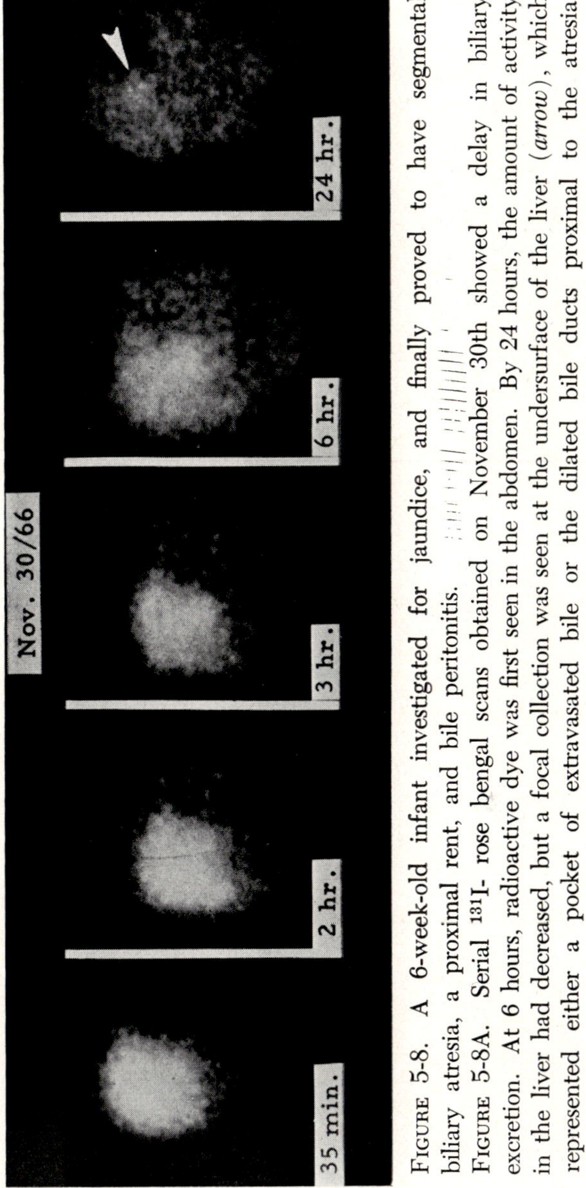

FIGURE 5-8. A 6-week-old infant investigated for jaundice, and finally proved to have segmental biliary atresia, a proximal rent, and bile peritonitis.
FIGURE 5-8A. Serial ^{131}I- rose bengal scans obtained on November 30th showed a delay in biliary excretion. At 6 hours, radioactive dye was first seen in the abdomen. By 24 hours, the amount of activity in the liver had decreased, but a focal collection was seen at the undersurface of the liver (*arrow*), which represented either a pocket of extravasated bile or the dilated bile ducts proximal to the atresia.

in detecting bile spill into the abdominal cavity. Figure 5-7 is a series obtained from an 80 year old male with carcinoma of the bile ducts. A T-tube was inserted into the right hepatic duct as a palliative procedure to relieve the obstructive jaundice. Post-operatively, the patient developed a high fever. The bilirubin

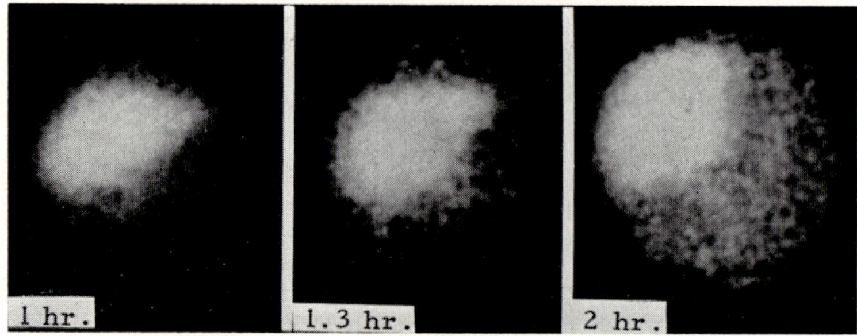

FIGURE 5-8B. On December 13th, a repeat radionuclide examination was performed. At this time, the infant had clinically detactable ascites. A uniform distribution of ^{131}I- rose bengal was observed throughout the abdomen suddenly at 2 hours, and apparently dissolved in the ascitic fluid.

was 4.3 mg per cent, and the alkaline phosphatase was rising. Serial ^{131}I- rose bengal scans showed a reduction in concentration of activity in the right lobe relative to the left at 1 and 4 hours. However, at 24 hours, there was an apparent reversal of the situation. Radioactive material was also demonstrated in the transverse colon. The initial impression was a blocked T-tube, but on inspection it proved to be patent. A bile leak was then suspected, and it was confirmed at laparotomy, where the bile was noted to be collecting over the surface of the right lobe.

Another example of bile peritonitis was observed in a six week old infant investigated for jaundice. On November 30th, about 50 microcuries ^{131}I- rose bengal was administered via

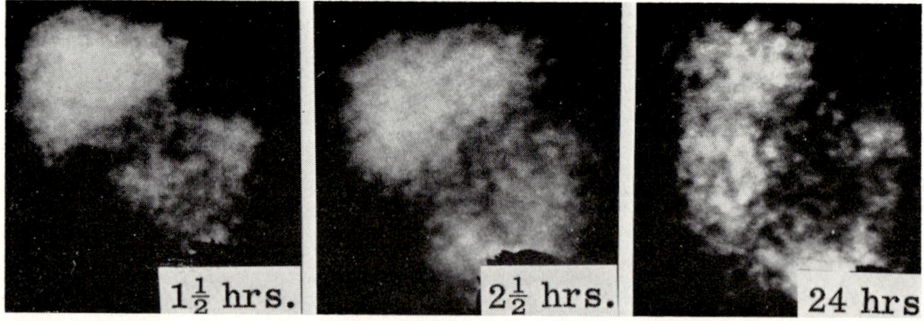

FIGURE 5-8C. Following a choledocho-duodenostomy for a segmental biliary atresia at the junction of the common hepatic and cystic ducts, a near normal ^{131}I- rose bengal scan sequence was obtained.

venapuncture, and a prompt uptake by the liver was noted (Fig. 5-8A). At 6 hours and 24 hours, radioactive dye was seen in the abdomen, but there was also a focal collection adjacent to the undersurface of the liver (*arrow*). The infant deteriorated clinically and developed an ascites. A repeat study on December 13th (Fig. 5-8B) showed a uniform distribution of activity throughout the abdomen at 2 hours, obviously not in the bowel, but dissolved in the ascitic fluid. At laparotomy, a biliary atresia at the junction of the common hepatic and cystic ducts was found, with a tear just proximal to it. In retrospect, although there was no clinical suspicion of a peritonitis on November 30th, there was obviously a bile leak, and the collection at the undersurface of the liver either represented a dilated duct system or a pocket of extravasated bile. Neither of these features was appreciated when the scans were first interpreted. A choledocho-duodenostomy was performed and the infant made an uneventful recovery. The series taken one month after surgery is depicted in Figure 5-8C, and it shows a near normal sequence of liver uptake and excretion.

DIFFERENTIATION OF INTRAHEPATIC DISEASE AND EXTRAHEPATIC BILIARY ATRESIA IN INFANTS

Obstructive jaundice in the neonatal stage of life is a perplexing diagnostic problem (6, 7, 8). Liver function studies and fecal pigment determinations are usually inconclusive, and this has led many authors to think that a surgical exploration is the only way to firmly establish an early diagnosis. Placing the infant under observation for a few months to determine whether the icterus will subside, as might be expected in neonatal hepatitis, or persist, which demands laparotomy, runs the risk of inducing a secondary cirrhosis in a situation that might have been subject to curative surgery.

Brent and Geppert (9) followed the excretion of 1 to 4 microcuries ^{131}I- rose bengal in thirteen infants with neonatal hepatitis and biliary atresia. In 4 cases of proved biliary atresia, the 72-hour stool collection recovered about 2% of the administered dose. The minimum 72-hour fecal excretion in the neonatal hepatitis group was 4.4%. One patient in the latter group was studied twice one month apart, and the value increased from 4.4% to 17.2%.

A similar investigation was reported by Ghadimi and Sass-Kortsak (10). They used 1 to 10 mg of rose bengal containing 1 microcurie of ^{131}I, and assayed the 72-hour stool collection. In 3 normal infants, 70 to 90% of the administered dose was recovered. The lowest fecal activity recovered in the group of six infants with neonatal hepatitis was 10.5%. A maximum value of 5% was obtained in four infants with biliary atresia. In a fifth infant, the fecal excretion was 51% following surgical correction of an atretic-duct. In one case of biliary atresia, 5% of the dose appeared in the stool when 10 mg of dye-carrier was added, but only 2.2% was excreted when the carrier-dose was only 1 mg of dye. The authors conclude that when a fecal excretion of 10% or more of the administered dose is obtained it should be regarded as evidence of incomplete biliary obstruction, which is incompatible with a diagnosis of biliary atresia. Less than 5% excretion makes surgical exploration mandatory, and although the occasional patient with complete biliary shut-down, but patent extrahepatic ducts, will be explored, it is better to err in this direction than to deny the possible advantages of surgical correction.

Becker and Hoeffler (11) describe three cases of biliary atresia with 72-hour stool collections of 3.6, 5.4 and 8.2% of the administered ^{131}I- rose bengal, and as a result feel that any value less than 10% justifies a laparotomy.

Sharp *et al.* (12) employed a 48-hour stool collection and injected 1 microcurie per kilogram ^{131}I- rose bengal. They analyzed the results of four groups of infants. The five controls passed 75 to 97% of the administered dose. 2.4 to 6.5% was collected from 10 neonates with extrahepatic biliary atresia, whereas 6 patients with neonatal obstructive intrinsic liver disease had 48-hour stool collections containing 14 to 73% of the dose. The last group of 14 infants consisted of a variety of liver dysfunctions due to histiocytosis X, plasma cell hepatitis, portal cirrhosis, diphenylhydantoin hepatitis and Aldrich syndrome. A range of 14 to 95% ^{131}I- rose bengal stool recovery was obtained.

A summary of the results achieved with an intravenous

injection of [131]I- rose bengal and assay of stool recovery in infants is given in the following table:

Report	Condition	Number of Patients	% of [131]I Recovered in 72 hr. Stool Collection
Brent and Geppert[9]	Biliary atresia	4	≤ 2
	Neonatal hepatitis	9	≥ 4.4
Ghadimi and Sass-Kortsak[10]	Normal	3	≥ 70
	Biliary atresia	4	≤ 5
	Neonatal hepatitis	6	≥ 10.5
Becker and Hoeffler[11]	Biliary atresia	3	≤ 8.2
Sharp *et al.*[12]	Normal	5	≥ 75*
	Biliary atresia	10	≤ 6.5*
	Neonatal hepatitis	20	≥ 14*

* 48-hour stool collection

Rosenthall (2), and Rosenthall and Silverberg (13) have adopted the use of serial [131]I- rose bengal liver and abdomen scans to observe the presence or absence of excretion into the bowel. A 50 microcurie scanning dose is employed, and the infants are medicated for three consecutive days with Lugol's solution to block the uptake by the thyroid of released radio-iodine. Scans can be obtained as frequently as desired, but 24, 48 and 72-hour views are mandatory. The study can be terminated before 72 hours if radioactivity in the gut is definitely established. Thirteen infants have thus far been studied—3 controls, 4 biliary atresias, and 6 with neonatal hepatitis.

Figure 5-9 is a sequence from the normal infant 10 months

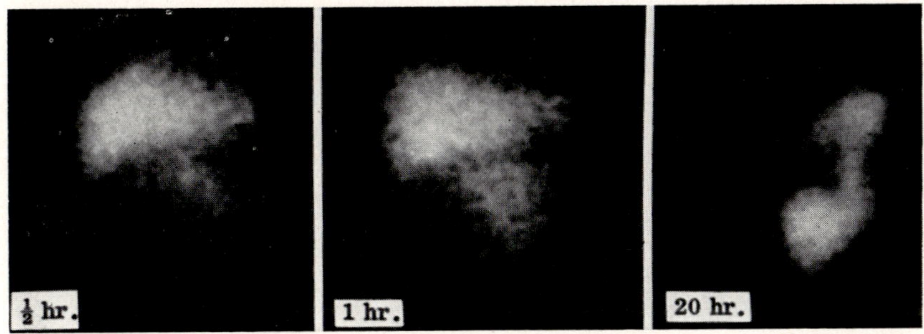

FIGURE 5-9.   A normal [131]I- rose bengal sequence in a 10 month old infant. Biliary excretion is seen at a half hour. At 20 hours, the liver is completely drained, and the radioactive dye is confined to the colon.

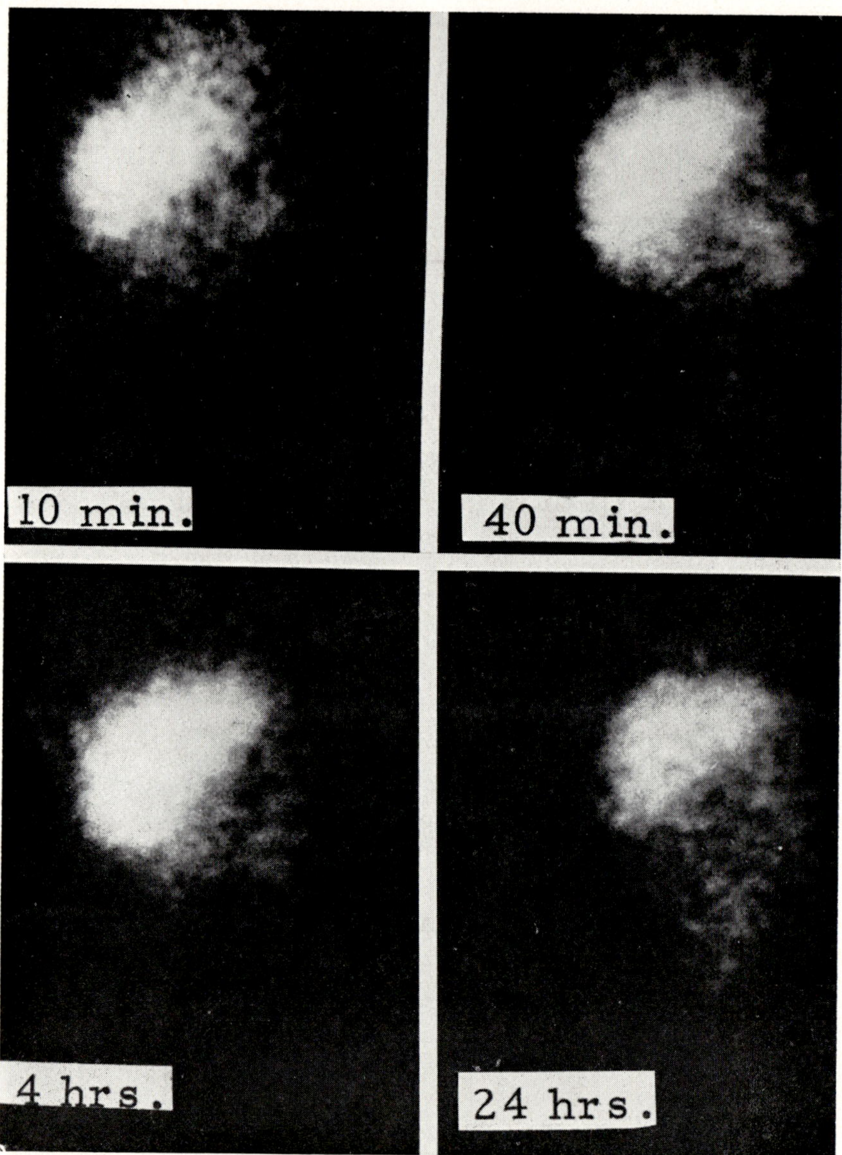

FIGURE 5-10.   A 5-week-old infant with neonatal hepatitis and obstructive blood chemistries. The ^{131}I- rose bengal studies showed delayed excretion into the gut, and was only definitely identified at 24 hours to establish biliary patency. Extra hepatic activity observed at 40 minutes and 4 hours most likely represents renal concentration.

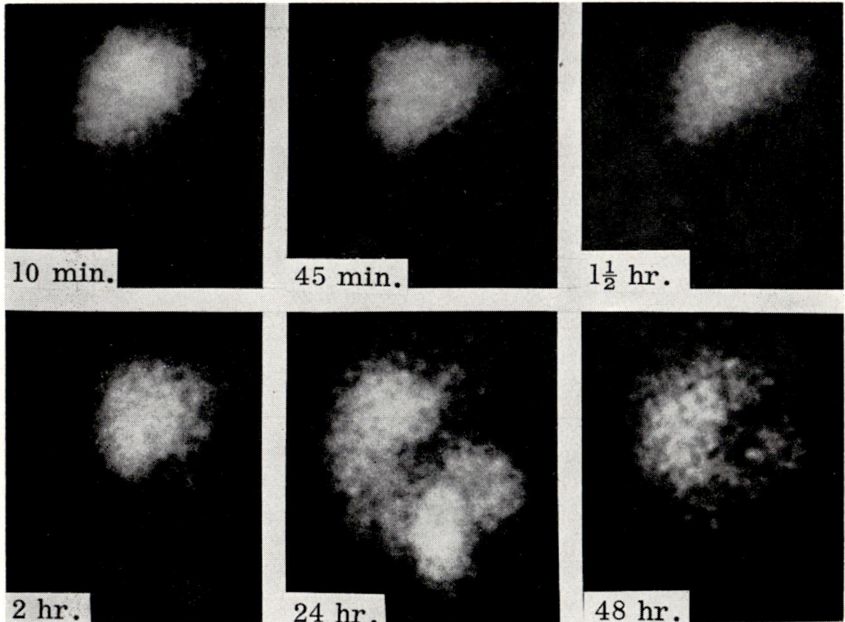

FIGURE 5-11.   Septic hepatitis was the final diagnosis in this 6 week old infant. Serial [131]I- rose bengal scans showed a prompty uptake at 10 minutes, but there was no appreciable excretion until 24 hours to rule out biliary atresia. At 48 hours, most of the bowel activity was lost with defecation, but residual radio-dye is observed in the liver.

of age. Excretion into the intestines is present as early as a half hour after the radioactive rose bengal was given. At 20 hours, the liver is no longer visualized, and the activity is confined to the left hemicolon.

A 5-week-old female neonate with obstructive blood and urine chemistries is illustrated in Figure 5-10. There is no conclusive evidence of intestinal bile entry at 4 hours, as the activity seen could be in the kidneys. However, at 24 hours, radioactive material is scattered throughout the abdomen, even though most of it still resides in the liver. A 48-hour study in an infant with a diagnosis of septic hepatitis is seen in Figure 5-11. No bile excretion is observed until 24 hours. At 48 hours, most of it had probably disappeared with defecation, but some activity is still visualized in the bowel and liver.

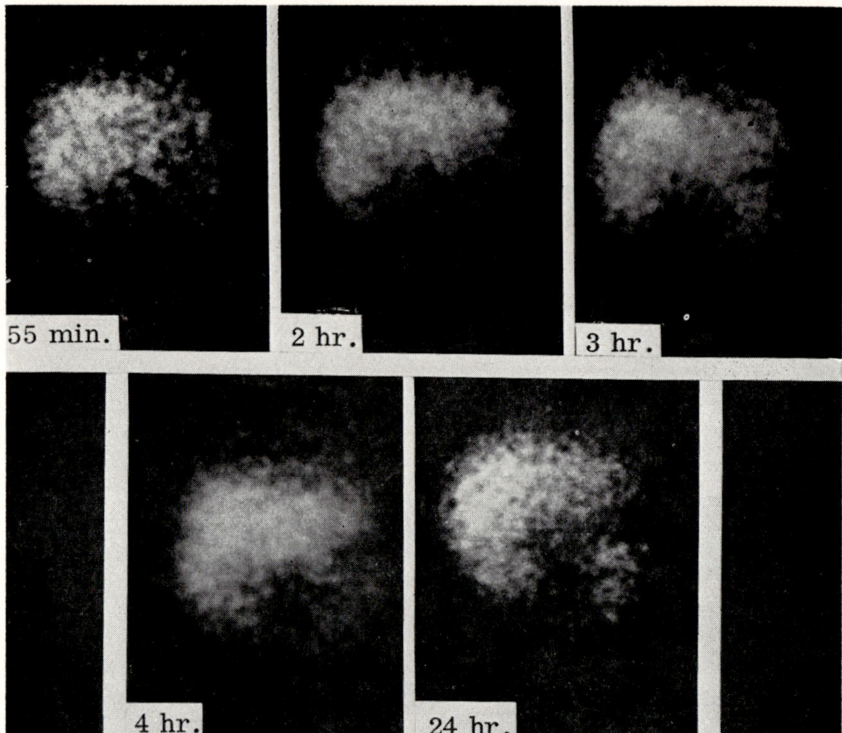

FIGURE 5-12. A proved case of biliary atresia showing no excretion into the bowel in 24 hours with the radioactive rose bengal series. The kidneys are well seen from 3 hours onward.

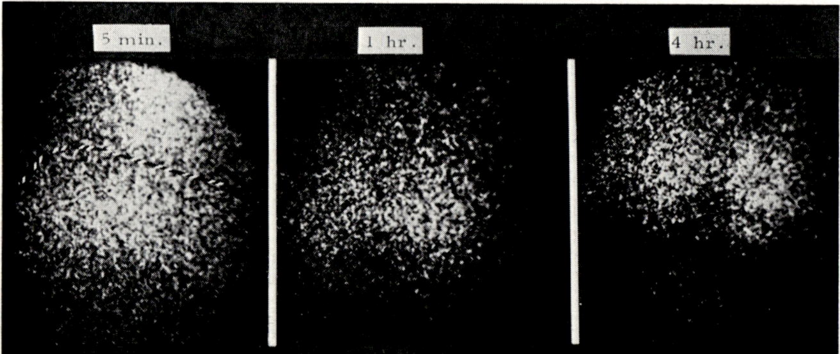

FIGURE 5-13. This 2½-year-old child had proved biliary atresia. Serial ^{131}I-rose bengal scans showed radioactivity in the cardiac blood pool and liver area at 5 minutes. At 1 hour, the cardiac blood cleared and the liver concentration was not well defined. By 4 hours, the bulk of the radioactivity was confined to the kidneys. This differs from the sequence of events obtained in neonates. (Reproduced, courtesy the *Am. J. Roentgenol., Rad.*

A proved case of biliary atresia in a 6-week-old infant is depicted in Figure 5-12, which contains selected scans from a radioactive rose bengal sequence. Activity is confined to the hepar and kidneys alone. A rather unique finding in a 2½ year old male child with biliary atresia is observed in Figure 5-13. Instead of the usual confinement of the test agent to the liver for several days as encountered with neonates, it is seen in the liver region only at 5 minutes. At 1 hour, the liver cannot be identified, and the tracer seems to be accumulating in the kidneys. Renal outlines crystalize at 4 hours and appear to be the only site of radioactivity. The reason for this phenomenon in the older biliary atretic is not readily explained.

There was one case in this series where no bile flow was visualized at 24 hours, and the examination was terminated with a radionuclide diagnosis of biliary atresia. A liver biopsy was somewhat confusing at the time, but several months later the infant improved, and a repeat radioactive rose bengal study showed excretion within 24 hours. This must be labelled as a false-positive, but perhaps a correct diagnosis would have been reached if the initial examination was extended to 72 hours.

In summary, the observation of radioactivity in bowel rules out biliary atresia, but the absence of it is not necessarily diagnostic of the condition.

A comparison of the absorbed radiation doses for ^{131}I- rose bengal and 1 minute of abdominal fluoroscopy are tabulated below (10):

Area	1 Microcurie* ^{131}I- Rose Bengal (millirads)	50 Microcuries* Scanning Dose of ^{131}I- Rose Bengal (millirads)	1 Minute of† Abdominal Fluoroscopy (millirads)
Whole body	5	250	450
Liver	340	17,000	3,000
Gonads	33	1,650	450

* Assuming an infant weight of 4 kg, and a liver mass of 140 gm. Figures are based on complete extrahepatic obstruction, complete dissociation of ^{131}I, a biological half-life of 3 days, and a circulation of 5% of the total radioactivity at any one time.
† Technical factors of 60 kev, 2 mm aluminum half-value layer, and a tabletop exposure of 3 roentgens per minute.

The scanning dose of 50 microcuries is somewhat high, but not entirely objectionable considering that 1 minute of abdominal fluoroscopy is a very conservative estimate of how much infants receive in practice. With rapid imaging devices, such as the gamma-ray scintillation camera or large crystal rectilinear scanners, the dose of ^{131}I- rose bengal may be halved to 25 microcuries. The technique does obviate stool collection, and contamination of the stool with urine which can offset the results of the assay.

BIBLIOGRAPHY

1. BURKE, G., AND HALKO, ARLENE: Dynamic clinical studies with radioisotopes and the scintillation camera. *J.A.M.A., 198*:6, 1966.
2. ROSENTHALL, L.: The application of colloidal radiogold and radioiodinated rose bengal in hepatobiliary disease. *Am. J. Roentgenol., Rad. Therap. & Nucl. Med., 101*:561, 1967.
3. EYLER, W. R., SCHUMAN, B. M., DUSAULT, L., AIKENS, N. R., AND HINSON, R. E.: Rose bengal-I^{131} liver scan. An aid to the differential diagnosis of jaundice. *J.A.M.A., 194*:990, 1965.
4. EYLER, W. R., SCHUMAN, B. M., DUSAULT, L. A., AND HINSON, R. E.: The radioiodinated rose bengal liver scan as an aid in the differential diagnosis of jaundice. *Am. J. Roentgenol., Rad. Therap. & Nucl. Med., 94*:469, 1965.
5. SHEHADI, W. H.: Practical applications of liver scanning. *Radiology, 86*:726, 1966.
6. NORRIS, W. J., AND HAYS, D. M.: Problems in diagnosis associated with obstructive neonatal jaundice. *Am. J. Surg., 94*:321, 1957.
7. SILVERBERG, M., CRAIG, I., AND GELLIS, S. S.: Problems in the diagnosis of biliary atresia—A review and consideration of histologic criteria. *Am. J. Dis. Child., 99*:574, 1960.
8. BENNETT, D. E.: Problems in neonatal obstructive jaundice. *Pediatrics, 33*:735, 1964.
9. BRENT, R. L., AND GEPPERT, L. J.: The use of radioactive rose bengal in the evaluation of infantile jaundice. *A.M.A. J. Dis. Child., 98*:270, 1959.
10. GHADIMI, H., AND SASS-KORTSAK, A.: Evaluation of the radioactive rose bengal test for the differential diagnosis of obstructive jaundice in infants. *New Eng. J. Med., 265*:351, 1961.
11. BECKER, F. B., AND HOEFFLER, D. F.: The radioactive rose bengal test. Its value in the diagnosis of extrahepatic biliary atresia in young infants. *Clin. Pediatrics, 3*:714, 1964.
12. SHARP, H. L., KRIVIT, W., AND LOWMAN, J. T.: The diagnosis of complete extrahepatic obstruction by rose bengal I^{131}. *Pediatrics, 70*:46, 1967.
13. ROSENTHALL, L., AND SILVERBERG, M.: Unpublished data.

INDEX